FOR THOSE IN NEED . . .

This cookbook by Pat & Ed Krimmel is an extension of the information presented in their book, THE LOW BLOOD SUGAR HANDBOOK.

They have done their best in THE LOW BLOOD SUGAR COOK-BOOK to help you prepare the best for your best. It is a very special collection of recipes for the whole world to enjoy. The authors are happy and thankful for all the help these recipes have given them and now want to share the benefits with you.

These recipes are tasty to the palate without being dangerous to the body's chemistry. They are presented in a format that allows for easy reading and preparation. Special effort was taken to design a format pleasant to the eye and easy on the spirit

Ordinary snacks to delightflul gourmet dishes are presented along with everything you need to know to prepare foods to help stabilize your blood sugar. No refined carbohydrates (white flour and sugar) or artifical sweetners are used. Rather, only whole grain flours are used and small amounts of fruits and fruit juices when sweetners are needed.

Eliminating refined carbohydrates from your diet helps eliminate many of the symptoms of functional hypoglycemia such as headaches, sensitivity to bright lights and loud noises, constant feeling of tiredness, sleeping problems, mood swings, overweight, etc.

Even though THE LOW BLOOD SUGAR COOKBOOK was written primarily for low blood sugar sufferers (hypoglycemics), it is equally beneficial to diabetics and weight watchers. In fact, this cookbook is for everyone interested in eating correctly so as to have a healthy, productive and creative life and spirit.

> A book for those who are learning to enjoy
> riding in the wagon for a change, rather
> than always having to push or pull it.
>
> Don't feel exstressive!
> Balance your body chemistry.

WE DEDICATE THIS BOOK

To the Lord and all his loving creatures who desire a healthy, productive and creative life and spirit.

To our Parents for being the fountainhead of our lives and spirits.

> Pat & Ed Krimmel

ACKNOWLEDGEMENTS

Roa Pattela, thank you for being supportive in everyway along the way.

Stephanie Barrett, thank you for all your time and support in getting us up and flying with our word proccessor.

Frank Smith, thank you for your everlasting patience and help.

Betty Aukstikalnes, thank you for our day in the sun and your tireless effort.

Jim Duffy, thank you for being you and again coming to our aid with your always dependable skill.

Joe Ruggiero, your kind support got us through the hi-tech and into print. Thank you.

RECIPE 716
serves all

Measure and prepare for one day at a time,
plan with a sense of flexibility
> Pour forth fresh faith, thoughts, and feelings
> with a pure heart and mind.
>> Offer time, thought and consideration to all
>> without waste or thought of reward.
>>> After works are done,
>>> shop for enjoyment and fun with deep laughter
>>> not excitement or danger. Mix carefully!

Reading and writing are dangerous
but clear thought and health are required,
check for freshness and motives.
> When preparing, taste often.
> When serving, be sure to use finest settings.
>> If need, ask for help but always give daily thanks.
>> Do not fear the Lord or yourself.
>>> Life's greatest strength is in gentleness.
>>> Seek and serve with caution for greatest purpose.

> Ed Krimmel

Extend yourself, the Lord is with you.
> Dr. Robert Schuller; The Hour of Power

THE
LOW BLOOD SUGAR
COOKBOOK

Sugarless Cooking For Everyone . . .

Patricia T. Krimmel
Edward A. Krimmel

Art & Design Editor
Charles A. Krimmel

FRANKLIN PUBLISHERS

Box 1338
Bryn Mawr, PA 19010

This cookbook is not meant to be a substitute in any way for proper medical care. It is a collection of recipes for functional hypoglycemics and others interested in eating foods which do not contain refined carbohydrates. It must be remembered that eating is the means by which we keep the cells in our bodies alive. The nutrients in the foods we eat are the nutrients which our cells must use to function and survive. Our cells will be only as healthy as the foods we eat and the foods we eat will be only as healthy as the nutrients in those foods.

Library of Congress Catalog No 85-80481

ISBN 0-916503-01-1   Printed in the U.S.A

CONTENTS

RECIPE 29
serves all

For human growth collect:
  great amounts of time, space and love.
Add:
  just the right amount of security and safety.
Permit as little:
  government intervention as possible into your
  life.
Safeguard against:
  non-elected persons in authority.
Trust your life and loved ones:
  to no one except the Lord.
Remember and seek:
  the peace that lives in silence, truth and joy.
Always season life with:
  achievements and plans regardless of potential
  monetary rewards.
Be enthusiastic:
  in your efforts.
Be concerned with:
  time and its applications, remain an effective
  time binder.
For savoring:
  face each day as a gift anew for the purpose of
  problem solving.
You are:
  the author of each day's worth, spend it wisely.
Give thanks.

      Ed Krimmel

The Krimmel Health Key:
  Eat high quality foods in small quantities frequently.

INTRODUCTION

The traditional functional hypoglycemic diet has been high protein (meat, fish, poultry, eggs and cheese) and low carbohydrate foods. Medical science has shown that too much protein and fat are detrimental to one's overall health. Therefore you should be following a low protein, high complex carbohydrate and low fat food ethic. Your daily calorie intake should be comprised of:

  50-65% from carbohydrate
  10-12% from protein
  20-30% from fat, visible and invisible, mostly unsaturated fat

Some studies have found that even though simple carbohydrates (sugar, white flour, fruit, etc) usually cannot be tolerated by hypoglycemics, many hypoglycemics can tolerate and enjoy complex carbohydrates (whole grains, legumes, vegetables, etc).

Some complex carbohydrates can be combined to form complete proteins, thereby reducing the needed amount of what is normally thought of as the "only" protein foods. Therefore we have included many whole grains and legumes in our recipes. The high fiber in these and other foods also helps starches be absorbed slowly into the blood stream thereby giving a gradual blood sugar rise rather than causing it to rise rapidly.

Since each person's body chemistry is different, especially hypoglycemics, foods that may be beneficial for one person may not be for another. Keeping this in mind we have endeavored to offer a variety of recipes to complement the needs of a variety of individuals.

Why did we write The Low Blood Sugar Cookbook? Because most recipes use white flour, sugar and other refined carbohydrates that are detrimental to a low blood sugar sufferer, our recipes avoid these substances. In addition we have not used artifical sweeteners, food additives or artifical colorings and flavorings in any of the recipes.

Why are refined carbohydrates detrimental? One theory is that low blood sugar sufferers secrete too much insulin from their pancreas when they eat refined carbohydrates, thus lowering their blood sugar (glucose) too rapidly, which produces an array of unpleasant symptoms (mood swings, fatigue, headaches, blurred vision, irritability, etc.)

Why do these symptoms appear when the blood sugar is too low? The cells of the body use glucose for energy. If the level of glucose is too low there is not enough energy for the cells to function efficiently. When cells don't function efficiently, symptoms appear telling us something is wrong. Most cells of the body can utilize fat and protein, in the absence of glucose, for energy. However the cells of the brain and retina of the eye can use only glucose for energy and need a constant and sufficient supply to function efficiently. When the cells of the brain and eyes aren't receiving enough energy, is it any wonder that symptoms appear!

Low blood sugar is a controllable condition. But you need more than just a cookbook. For a complete and comprehensive discussion of low blood sugar, its effects and solution, buy and use our LOW BLOOD SUGAR HANDBOOK. (See order form in back of book.)

God bless, and we love you too.

Pat & Ed Krimmel

PIZZA

Light! I was being pulled out of my box. I started to sweat. No, it wasn't sweat. Oh no, I was defrosting! I looked around and saw my five brothers and two sisters, they all looked pale and hopeless.

Then without any warning we were flung into another bigger box. Only instead of being cold, it was HOT! The moment I touched the bottom, my backside started to sizzle. The heat was slowly creeping through my breading, it was getting to the cheese. It was onto the sauce and I was bubbling!

I started to feel numb so I took some time to look around. There were about three other pizzas around me. What's that? It was a sharp buzz. Then it stopped. All of a sudden I was bathed in light.

I was taken out and rushed to a table. Oh no, there's five people at this table! "We will be gone in a second", I heard Chrisy, my younger sister, say as she was being picked up. Then all of a sudden it attacked me from behind. The hand grabbed violently and started pulling me upward. My toes and fingers started being stretched and pulled. Then they snapped free and twanged up. One of my fingers had a little bit of sauce on it. When it snapped back, it hit the guy holding me right on the nose. Then he folded me in half and started stuffing his face. It was disgusting. It didn't hurt much because he was the kind of guy who when he gets his hands on food, it doesn't last long

By
Charles Krimmel

GENERAL INFORMATION

An important and simple aspect of getting your blood sugar stabilized is eating what is best for your blood sugar. Removing refined carbohydrates (white flour, sugars and processed foods) from your diet is the first step and then adding more complex carbohydrates (vegetables, whole grains, legumes, nuts, and seeds), is what we are trying to help you do in this cookbook.

When first beginning to stabilize your blood sugar you shouldn't eat any type of flour products. Gradually you will begin adding whole grains and whole grain products. (see our book, THE LOW BLOOD SUGAR HANDBOOK for a specfic under-standing of the low blood sugar food program)

One of the best grains for a hypoglycemic is oats. Unlike the wheat which is made into white flour, oats go through the milling process retaining most of their nutrients. Only the hull is removed leaving most of the bran, endosperm and germ. This leaves the oats rich in protein, vitamins and minerals. Oats not only have the highest protein content of the grains but also have the highest quality protein. This is the reason we have tried to use oats and oat flour rather than just whole wheat flour in as many baked goods an possible. Also the incidence of oat allergy is much lower than wheat allergy.

Oat flour can be bought in a health food store or very easily made at home as needed by grinding rolled oats or oat flakes in a blender. I have found that some commerical oat flour must be shifted where as what you make doesn't need to be. Besides using in baked goods, oat flour can be used to thicken gravies if you must thicken them.

Try other whole grain flours such as rye, buck wheat, Ezekiel (combination of whole grains, beans and lentils) and triticale.

For sweeteners we have used unsweetened fruit juices, frozen fruit juice concentrates and liquid fruit concentrates. You can try different juices if you desire. We have stayed away from artifical sweeteners because of possible unknown side effects and the false sense of security they give.

Soybean and its products have an excellent combination of protein and carbohydrate which make them very helpful to hypoglycemics. Tofu, soybean curd provides protein, calcium, phosphorus, potassium and some B and E vitamins. It is ideal to use in place of meat in dishes where it will absorb flavors of the foods with which it is cooked. A small amount of soy flour can be added to baked goods to increase their nutritional value.

Chocolate and cocoa are no no's for hypoglycemics, however for those who think they can't live without them there is a food somewhat similar. Carob has the same general appearance as chocolate and has its own light, slightly milk-chocolatey flavor but it does not contain caffeine. Because of its own natural sweetness you can buy it without sugar having been added. As a bonus it provides some nutrition in the form of A and B vitamins and some calcium, potassium, iron and pectin. It is available in powder and chips, just be sure to read the label for added sugar. Even if sugar has not been added, don't over indulge, remember, too much natural sugar can also cause problems.

When eating, it is best to think about what foods will make the cells in our body function best rather than what foods taste best. It's a question of, are you going to control your body's chemistry or is the tip of your tongue going to control your body's chemistry and subsquently your personal well-being? Well???

Here's a tidbit of information for those who say they have poor self control regarding sweets or whatever they crave to eat. When the blood sugar level falls, the first area of the brain to be affected is the neocortex. And guess what the neocortex controls! It controls the self control center. However if the blood sugar is kept at a stable level then there can be much better control of what we eat and how often. Talk about a handshaking relationship in a darkened room!

"Turkey Sam"

There once was this turkey named Sam,
Who sat eating Thanksgiving ham.
He thought with a grin
As he wiped off his chin,
"What a sly old fellow, I am!"

"I outsmarted the farmer, it's true;
And he'd be really mad if he knew
That I lost all that weight
Before the big date
So I'd enjoy Thanksgiving, too!"

By
Judy Robinson, Poet
Hollis, Oklahoma

ENTREES

The following entrees (main dishes) range from traditional meat and chicken dishes to not-so-familiar tofu dishes. Some recipes include rice or potatoes which you might think should not be eaten because of their high starch content. It is for sure that a hypoglycemic just beginning to get stabilized should not eat these but one whose body's chemistry is stable may enjoy a moderate serving.

Other entrees do not contain meat of any type and you may wonder how you will be eating sufficient protein. Grains, nuts & seeds (sesame, sunflower) and legumes (beans, peas and lentils) all contain protein and when combined or served together make a complete protein. This is a perfect example of not having to eat meat to get suffficient complete protein.

Amino acids are the building blocks of proteins. There are 22 amino acids of which nine cannot be made by our bodies and therefore we must get them from the foods we eat. These nine are needed simultaneously and in the right proportion for the protein to be beneficial. Subsquently they are referred to as the essential amino acids.

Grains, nuts, seeds and legumes have the 9 essential amino acids in varying degrees. Therefore you can eat just these to get sufficient protein providing you eat them in the proper combinations.

The best combinations are: grains with legumes, seeds with legumes or grains with a milk product. To a lesser degree, grains with seeds, seeds with a milk product or legumes with a milk product give you a complete protein.

An excellent legume protein is tofu which comes from soy beans. It is high in protein and very versatile.

For a detailed and specific understanding of using complementing foods to give a complete protein, read DIET FOR A SMALL PLANET by Frances Moore Lappe.

We find a salad and whole grain muffins excellent compliments to quiche dishes. Quiche recipes are especially flexible in allowing for the chef's individual creativity. A variety of vegetables and/or herbs may be used to express your individual taste and desire.

NO CRUST QUICHE
serves 4-6

Ingredients:
eggs 3
salt ⅛ tsp.
nutmeg, dash
jarlsberg cheese 1 cup
fresh spinach 1 cup

milk or light cream 1 cup
dry mustard ¼ tsp.
onion ½
cheddar cheese ½ cup

Preparation:
Beat together:
   3 eggs
   1 cup warm milk or light cream
   ⅛ tsp. salt
   ¼ tsp. dry mustard
   dash of nutmeg

Add:
   1 cup shredded jarlsberg cheese
   ½ cup shredded cheddar cheese
   1 cup chopped fresh spinach

Sauté and add to above:
   ½ onion, cut into thin slices

Mix well
Pour into 8 inch glass pie plate

Bake 45 minutes at 350° or until set

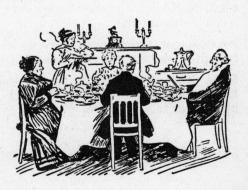

THREE CHEESE QUICHE
serves 6

Ingredients:

eggs 3
salt ¼ tsp.
Monterey Jack cheese 2 cups
chives 1 Tbs.

milk ½ cup
pepper ⅛ tsp.
cottage cheese ¾ cup
cream cheese 1 ½ oz

Preparation:

In small bowl, combine at low speed of electric mixer:
3 eggs
½ cup milk
¼ tsp. salt
⅛ tsp. pepper

Add and beat until thoroughly blended:
2 cups shredded Monterey Jack cheese
¾ cup cottage cheese
1 Tbs. chives
1 ½ oz. cream cheese, cut up

Pour into 9" glass pie plate
Bake at 350° for 25-30 minutes

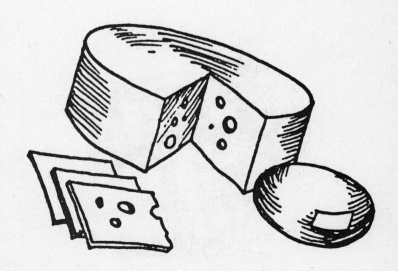

SHRIMP AND MUSHROOM QUICHE
serves 4-6

Ingredients:
mushrooms ¾ cup

green onion ⅓ cup

eggs 4

salt ¼ tsp.

shrimp 7 oz.

jarlsberg cheese ⅓ lb.

milk or half & half 1 ¾ cups

Preparation:
Sauté:

  ¾ cup sliced mushrooms

Combine in bowl:

  ¾ cup mushrooms

  7 oz. chopped shrimp

  ⅓ cup minced green onion

  ⅓ lb. shredded jarlsberg cheese

Spread mixture into 9 inch glass pie plate

Combine in bowl:

  4 eggs

  1 ¾ cups milk or half & half

  ¼ tsp. salt

Pour over cheese

Bake at 350° for 30 minutes or until set

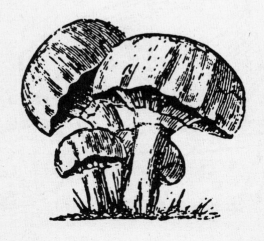

VEGETABLE QUICHE CASSEROLE
serves 6

Ingredients:
vegetable oil 2 Tbs.
garlic clove 1
broccoli 1 ½ cups
cauliflower 1 cup
eggs 6
salt ¼ tsp.
dried rosemary ¼ tsp.

onion 1
sweet red pepper 1
carrots ¾ cup
celery ¾ cup
sharp cheddar cheese 2 cups
dried basil ½ tsp.

Preparation:
Heat in skillet over medium heat:
 2 Tbs. vegetable oil
Add and sauté lightly:
 1 onion sliced thin
 1 garlic clove, minced
 1 sweet red pepper, minced
 1 ½ cups chopped broccoli
 ¾ cup sliced carrots
 1 cup chopped cauliflower
 ¾ cup chopped celery
Cover and steam for 3 minutes

Beat:
 6 eggs
Add and mix together:
 2 cups grated sharp cheddar cheese
 ¼ tsp. salt
 ½ tsp. dried basil, crushed
 ¼ tsp. dried rosemary, crushed
Add to vegetables mixture
Pour into oiled 1 ½ - 2 quart casserole

Bake 35 minutes at 325° or until lightly brown and set

TOFU PARMESAN
serves 6-8

Ingredients:
vegetable oil 4 Tbs.
mushrooms ¼ cup
zucchini ½ cup
celery ¼ cup
dried rosemary ¼ tsp.
salt ¼ tsp.
soy sauce 2 ⅓ Tbs.
oat flour ¼ cup
medium onions 2

garlic cloves 6
sweet red pepper ¼ cup
cut green beans ½ cup
broccoli ¼ cup
dried marjoram ¼ tsp.
tomato sauce 1 cup
egg 1
firm tofu 2 lb.
Parmesan cheese 1 cup

Preparation:
Heat in skillet over medium heat:
  2 Tbs. vegetable oil
Add and sauté for 1 minute:
  6 garlic cloves, chopped
Add and sauté for a few minutes:
  ¼ cup sliced mushrooms
  ¼ cup chopped sweet red pepper
  ½ cup chopped zucchini
  ½ cup cut green beans
  ¼ cup chopped celery
  ¼ cup chopped broccoli
Add:
  ¼ tsp. dried rosemary, crushed
  ¼ tsp. dried marjoram, crushed
  ¼ tsp. salt
  1 ½ cups water
  1 cup tomato sauce
  2 Tbs. soy sauce

Simmer a few minutes, remove from heat
Beat together in small dish:
  1 egg
  1 tsp. soy sauce
Pour onto plate:
  ¼ cup oat flour

Cut into 12 slices:
  2 lbs. firm tofu
Dip each slice of tofu into:
  egg mixture then flour

Brown tofu slices in:
  2 Tbs. vegetable oil
Place on bottom of large baking dish:
  12 slices of browned tofu
Place on top of tofu:
  2 medium onions, thinly sliced
Pour tomato sauce mixture over tofu and onions
Sprinkle on top:
  1 cup freshly grated parmesan cheese
Cover with lid or aluminum foil
Bake at 325° for ½ hour

Uncover, put holes in tofu with a fork
Bake 20 more minutes.

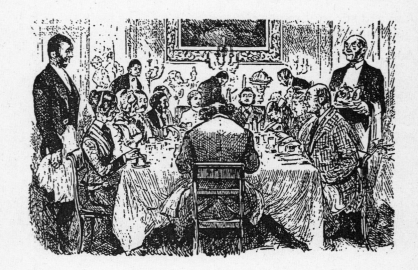

STIR FRIED TOFU AND VEGETABLES
serves 4-6

Ingredients:
vegetable oil 2 Tbs.
ginger ½ tsp.
cut green beans 1 cup
celery stalk 1
soy sauce 2 Tbs.
firm tofu ¾ lb.

garlic cloves 2
medium carrots 2
sweet red pepper 2
small onion 1
vinegar ⅔ Tbs.

Preparation:
Heat in large skillet or wok:
   2 Tbs. vegetable oil
Add and stir fry for 2 minutes:
   2 garlic cloves, minced
   ½ tsp. ginger
   2 medium carrots cut into thin slices
   1 cup cut green beans

Add and stir fry for another 2 minutes:
   2 sweet red peppers, cut into 1 inch pieces
   1 stalk celery cut into ½ inch pieces

Add and stir fry 1 minute:
   1 small onion, sliced

Add and stir together:
   2 Tbs. soy sauce
   ⅔ Tbs. vinegar
   ¾ lb. tofu, cut into ½ inch cubes

Cover and steam over low heat for 5-7 minutes
Serve immediately

NEAT, SWEET AND SOUR TOFU AND VEGETABLES
serves 4

Ingredients:

cider vinegar 1 Tbs.
soy sauce 2 Tbs.
pepper
medium onion 1
firm tofu ¾ lb
green pepper 1

unsweetened pineapple juice ¼ cup
ginger ¼-½ tsp.
vegetable oil 2 Tbs.
carrots 2
pineapple chunks with its juice ⅔ cup

Preparation:

Combine and set aside:
  1 Tbs. cider vinegar
  6 Tbs. water
  ¼ cup unsweetened pineapple juice
  2 Tbs. soy sauce
  ¼-½ tsp. ginger
  dash of pepper

Heat in wok or large skillet:
  2 Tbs. vegetable oil
Add and stir:
  1 medium onion, chopped
Add and stir:
  2 carrots, sliced thinly, diagonally
Add and stir until lightly brown:
  ¾ lb. tofu, cut into small chunks
Add and stir 1 minute:
  1 green pepper, chopped

Cover, reduce heat to medium
Cook until carrots partly cooked

Add:
  ⅔ cups pineapple chunks in own juice
  pineapple juice mixture
Cook covered for about 10 minutes
Serve over brown rice if desired

SUPER EGGPLANT PARMESAN
serves 6

Ingredients:

eggplant 1 ½ lb.
wheat germ 1 ¼ cups
pepper ½ tsp.
dried basil 1 tsp.
mozzarella cheese 1 lb.

eggs 2
salt ½ tsp.
tomato sauce 15 oz. can
dried oregano ½ tsp.
parmesan cheese ½ cup

Preparation:

Wash and cut crosswise into ½ inch slices:
   1 ½ lb. eggplant

Put in small dish and beat:
   2 eggs
Mix together on plate:
   1 ¼ cups wheat germ
   ½ tsp. salt
   ½ tsp. pepper

Dip eggplant slices into beaten eggs
Coat each slice with wheat germ
Place eggplant slices on plate and refrigerate ½ hour

Broil eggplant until sligthly brown on both sides

Combine and heat:
   1 15 oz. can tomato sauce
   1 tsp. dried basil, crushed
   ½ tsp. dried oregano, crushed
Spread small amount of tomato sauce on bottom of 12×8×2 inch
   baking dish

Layer on top of tomato sauce:
   ½ the eggplant slices
   ½ mozzarella cheese, sliced
   ½ remaining tomato sauce
   ¼ cup Parmesan cheese
Repeat layers

Bake at 350° for about 30 minutes or until bubbly

NO-DOUGH ZUCCHINI LASAGNA
serves 10-12

Ingredients:

large zucchinni 2 ½ -3 lbs.
eggs 4
oregano ½ tsp.
Parmesan cheese 1 cup
mozzarella cheese 1 lb.
salt

ricotta cheese 2 lbs
fresh parsley 2 Tbs
basil ½ tsp.
wheat germ 1 cup
spaghetti sauce (sugarless) 1 qt

Preparation:

Trim ends, slice into long thin slices:
 1 large zucchini 2 ½-3 lbs

Combine:
 2 lbs. ricotta cheese
 4 eggs, beaten
 2 Tbs. fresh chopped parsley
 ½ tsp. dried crushed oregano
 ½ tsp. dried crushed basil
 ½ cup Parmesan cheese
 ⅓ cup wheat germ

Spoon into a 9"x14"x2" baking dish:
 thin layer of spaghetti sauce(sugarless)
Sprinkle on sauce:
 ¼ cup wheat germ
Layer:
 ½ zucchini slices, side by side
 ½ ricotta cheese mixture
 ½ lb. grated mozzarella cheese
 ½ tomato sauce
Repeat layers

Combine and sprinkle over top:
 ½ cup Parmesan cheese
 ⅔ cup wheat germ
Bake at 350° for about 1 hour or until top browned
Let stand 15-20 minutes before serving

Ideal to cook a day ahead for convenience and purring flavor

Contributed by
Garfield

ZUCCHINI CASSEROLE
serves 4

Ingredients:
zucchini 2 cups

pepper ¼ tsp.

dried basil ½ tsp.

dill weed ¼ tsp.

fresh mushrooms ½ cup

Provolone cheese 4 slices

Parmesan cheese ⅓ cup

wheat germ ½ cup

parsley 1 tsp.

salt ¼ tsp.

small onion 1

eggs 2

large tomato 1

Preparation:
Mix together:
 2 cups chopped zucchini
 ½ cup wheat germ
 ¼ tsp. pepper
 1 tsp. parsley
 ½ tsp. dried basil, crushed
 ¼ tsp. salt
 ¼ tsp. dill weed
 1 small onion, chopped
 ½ cup fresh mushrooms, sliced
 2 eggs, beaten
Pour into shallow baking dish
Place on top:
 4 slices Provolone cheese

Place on top of cheese:
 1 large tomato, sliced
Sprinkle with:
 ⅓ cup Parmesan cheese

Bake at 350° for 30 minutes

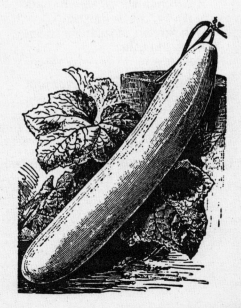

VEGETABLE NUT LOAF
serves 4-6

Ingredients:
medium onion 1
broccoli ½ cup
walnuts 1 cup
fresh parsley ½ cup
salt
rolled oats ¼ cup

cauliflower ½ cup
vegetable oil 1 Tbs.
cheddar cheese 1 cup
eggs 2
pepper

Preparation:
Heat in skillet:
   1 Tbs. vegetable oil
Add and sauté:
   1 medium onion, chopped
   ½ cup diced cauliflower
   ½ cup diced broccoli

Combine above with:
   1 cup finely chopped walnuts
   1 cup shredded sharp cheddar cheese
   ½ cup chopped fresh parsley
   2 eggs, beaten
   ¼ cup rolled oats
   salt and pepper to taste
Mix well

Place in well greased 8"x4" loaf pan

Bake at 350° for 25 minutes

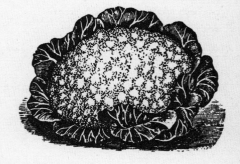

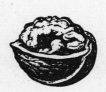

WALTER'S MOCK MEAT LOAF
serves 6-8

Ingredients:
eggs 4
Swiss cheese 2 cups
cooked brown rice 1 cup
fresh mushrooms ½ cup
garlic clove 1

cheddar cheese 2 cups
cashews 1 ½ cups
rolled oats ½ cup
onion 1
green pepper ½

Preparation:
Combine and mix well:
  4 eggs, beaten
  2 cups grated cheddar cheese
  2 cups grated Swiss cheese
  1 ½ cups chopped cashews
  1 cup cooked brown rice
  ½ cup rolled oats
  ½ cup chopped fresh mushrooms
  1 chopped onion
  1 garlic cloved, minced
  ½ green pepper, diced
Place in greased 9″ × 5″ × 3″ loaf pan
Bake at 350° for about 1 hour
Let stand 5-10 minutes before removing from pan

Pleasant when served with creamed mushrooms over slices of loaf

CREAMED MUSHROOMS

Ingredients:
butter ¼ cup
oat flour ¼ cup
pepper dash

fresh mushrooms 2 cups
salt ¼ tsp.
milk 2 cups

Preparation:
Melt in saucepan
  ¼ cup butter
Add and sauté for about 5 minutes:
  2 cups sliced fresh mushrooms
Stir in:
  ¼ cup oat flour
  ¼ tsp. salt
  dash pepper
Gradually stir in and cook till thickened, stirring constantly:
  2 cups milk

TOFU BURGERS
serves 8-10

Ingredients:

vegetable oil 1 Tbs.
celery stalk with leaves 1
tofu 1 ½ lb.
oat flour 2 Tbs.
salt ½ tsp.
garlic powder ¼ tsp.
tomato sauce ¼ cup

large onion ½
red pepper ½
egg 1
cooked brown rice 1 cup
soy sauce 2 Tbs.
oregano ½ tsp.

Preparation:

Sauté in 1 Tbs. vegetable oil:
  ½ large onion, chopped fine
  1 stalk celery with leaves, chopped fine
  ½ red pepper, chopped fine

Mash with fork:
  1 ½ lb. tofu
Add:
  1 egg, beaten
  2 Tbs. oat flour
  1 cup cooked brown rice
  ½ tsp. salt
  2 Tbs. soy sauce
  ¼ tsp. garlic powder
  ½ tsp. oregano, crushed
  ¼ cup tomato sauce
Add:
  sautéed vegetables
Mix well

Shape into patties

Bake at 350° for 30 minutes

CHICKEN CASSEROLE
serves 6

Ingredients:

carrots 2	celery stalks 2
onions 3	cut green beans 10 oz.
bay leaf 1	sweet red pepper ½ cup
cooked chicken 3 cups	chicken gravy 1 ½ cups
dried basil 1 tsp.	mushrooms ½ lb

Optional ingredients:

mash potatoes 2 cups	eggs 2
or	
oat flour 1 ½ cups	baking powder 3 tsp.
salt ¼ tsp.	eggs 2
milk ½ cup	vegetable oil ⅓ cup

Preparation:
Cook in 4 quart oven proof casserole until just tender:
    ¼ cup water
    2 carrots, chopped
    2 stalks celery, chopped
    3 onions, quartered
    10 oz. cut green beans
    1 bay leaf
    ½ cup chopped sweet red pepper

Add and mix together:
    3 cups diced cooked chicken
    1 ½ cups chicken gravy
    1 tsp. dried basil, crushed
    ½ lb. sliced mushrooms
    salt and pepper to taste

Bake at 350° for 30 minutes or until bubbly

Optional:
    Before baking:
        Mix together:
            2 cups mashed potatoes
            2 eggs beaten
        Spoon onto top of casserole ingredients
    Or

Mix together:
  1 ½ cups oat flour
  3 tsp. baking powder
  ¼ tsp. salt
Combine and add:
  2 eggs
  ½ cup milk
  ⅓ cup vegetable oil
Mix until just moistened
Spoon onto top of casserole ingredients

BARBECUED CHICKEN
serves 6-8

Ingredients:

fryer chickens 2
small onion 1
large bell pepper 1
salt ¼ tsp.
lemon juice 1 Tbs.
cayenne pepper ⅛ tsp.

oil 2 Tbs.
garlic clove 1
tomato sauce 8 oz.
vinegar 1 Tbs.
hot sauce ½ tsp.
basil leaves 1 tsp.

Preparation:
Skin chicken
Cut into serving pieces
Brush chicken with:
  2 Tbs. oil
Broil for 10 minutes
Combine and simmer for five minutes:
  1 small onion, diced
  1 garlic clove, crushed
  1 large bell pepper, diced
  8 oz. tomato sauce
  ¼ tsp. salt
  1 Tbs. vinegar
  1 Tbs. lemon juice
  ½ tsp. hot sauce
  ⅛ tsp. cayenne pepper
  1 tsp. basil leaves, crushed
Brush chicken with sauce

Bake at 350° for 1 hour

CHICKEN A LA KING
serves 4

Ingredients:

butter 3 Tbs.
onion 2 Tbs.
oat flour 2 Tbs.
milk 2 cups
red pimientos 2 Tbs.

green pepper 2 Tbs.
celery ¼ cup
salt ½ tsp.
cooked chicken 2 ½ cups
mushrooms ¾ cup

Preparation:

Melt in a skillet or stove top casserole:
  3 Tbs. butter
Add:
  2 Tbs. chopped green pepper
  2 Tbs. finely chopped onion
  ¼ cup diced celery
Sauté lightly

Stir in till well blended:
  2 Tbs. sifted oat flour
  ½ tsp. salt

Stir while adding:
  2 cups milk
Cook and stir until smooth and slightly thick

Add:
  2 ½ cups diced cooked chicken
  2 Tbs. chopped red pimientos
  ¾ cup sliced mushrooms
Stir until mixed
Heat thoroughly

Eat and enjoy as if a king.

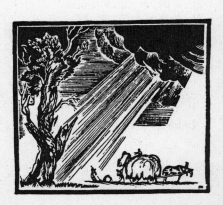

CHICKEN AND RICE
serves 4

Ingredients:

uncooked brown rice 1 cup
fresh mushrooms ¼ lb.
onion ½ cup
salt ¼ tsp.
garlic 1 clove
paprika

whole tomatoes 1 can (1 lb.)
celery 1 cup
dried basil ¾ tsp.
pepper ¼ tsp.
sweet red pepper 1
chicken 3 lb. fryer

Preparation:

Place in electric skillet:
    ¼ cup water
    1 cup uncooked brown rice
    1 can (1lb.) whole tomatoes, cut up
    ¼ lb. sliced fresh mushrooms
    1 cup chopped celery
    ½ cup chopped onion
    ¾ tsp. dried basil, crushed
    ¼ tsp. salt
    ¼ tsp. pepper
    1 clove garlic, minced
    1 sweet red pepper, chopped
Stir until mixed

Turn skillet on to 350°

Place on top of mixture:
    3 lb. chicken fryer, skinned and cut in serving pieces
Sprinkle on chicken:
    paprika
Put on lid

Bake for 50 - 60 minutes or until tender

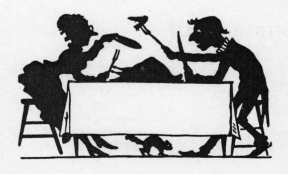

PERCH DIJON
serves 2-3

Ingredients:
frozen perch fillets 1 lb.
vegetable oil 1 Tbs.
apple juice 2 Tbs. (optional)
parsley 1 Tbs.
salt
wheat germ ¼ cup

onions 2 Tbs.
fresh mushrooms 1 ⅓ cup
Dijon mustard 1 Tbs.
marjoram, pinch
pepper
Swiss cheese 2 oz.

Preparation:
Heat in saucepan:
   1 Tbs. oil
Sauté till soft:
   2 Tbs. minced onion
Add, stir over high heat, 2 minutes
   1 ⅓ cups sliced mushrooms
Stir in:
   2 Tbs. water or apple juice
   1 Tbs. Dijon mustard
   1 Tbs. chopped parsley
   pinch marjoram
   salt & pepper to taste

Sprinkle in greased 7 ½"x11 ¾" baking dish:
   2 Tbs. wheat germ
Place frozen perch fillets in single layer
Spread over fish:
   mushroom mixture
   2 Tbs. wheat germ
   2 oz. grated Swiss cheese

Bake at 400° for about 25 minutes

COD MEDITERRANEAN
serves 2-3

Ingredients:
Frozen cod fillets 1 lb.
green pepper ¾
garlic clove 1
thyme ¼ tsp.
oregano ¼ tsp.
tomato paste 1 Tbs.

medium onion 1
olive oil 1 Tbs.
salt ⅛ tsp.
pepper ⅛ tsp.
chicken or vegetable stock ¼ cup
parsley 2 Tbs.

Preparation:
Place in lightly oiled casserole:
1 lb. frozen cod fillets, separated
Add, on top of fillets:
1 medium onion, sliced
¾ pepper, sliced

Combine and pour over fillets:
1 Tbs. olive oil
1 clove garlic, crushed
⅛ tsp. salt
¼ tsp. thyme
¼ tsp. oregano
⅛ pepper
¼ cup chicken or vegetable stock
1 Tbs. tomato paste

Bake at 425° for 25 minutes
Baste with sauce halfway thru cooking
Serve garnished with:
2 Tbs. chopped parsley

BAKED FLOUNDER
serves 2-3

Ingredients:

frozen flounder fillets 1 lb.   vegetable oil 1 Tbs.
salt   pepper
paprika   thyme ¼ tsp.
Swiss cheese 2 Tbs. (optional)

Preparation:
Place in greased baking dish:
1 lb. frozen flounder fillets, separated
Brush with:
1 Tbs. vegetable oil
Sprinkle with:
salt
paprika
pepper
¼ tsp. thyme
2 Tbs. grated Swiss cheese (optional)

Bake at 400° for 10-15 minutes

CRAB CASSEROLE
serves 4

Ingredients:
crab meat 1 lb.
small onion 1
salt ¼ tsp.
mayonnaise ⅓ cup
fresh parmesan cheese ⅓ cup

small sweet red pepper 1
celery ¾ cup
pepper
wheat germ ⅓ cup
butter 2 tsp.

Preparation:
Combine:
   1 lb. crab meat
   1 small sweet red pepper, chopped
   1 small onion, chopped
   ¾ cup chopped celery
   ¼ tsp. salt
   pepper to taste
   ⅓ cup mayonnaise
Place mixture in 2 quart casserole

Mix together:
   ⅓ cup wheat germ
   ⅓ cup shredded fresh parmesan cheese
Sprinkle over top of crab mixture
Dot with:
   2 tsp. butter

Bake at 350° for 40 minutes

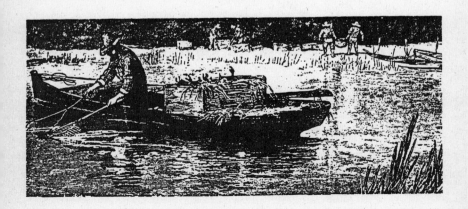

CRAB IMPERIAL
serves 4

Ingredients:
oat flour 1 ⅓ Tbs.
salt ¼ tsp.
butter 1 ⅔ Tbs.
egg yolks 2

dry mustard 1 tsp.
cayenne pepper dash
milk 1 cup
crab meat 12 oz.

Preparation:
Mix together:
  1 ⅓ Tbs. oat flour
  1 tsp dry mustard
  ¼ tsp. salt
  dash cayenne pepper

Melt in small saucepan:
  1 ⅔ Tbs. butter
Stir in:
  flour mixture
  ¾ cup milk
Let come to boil
Cook for 5 minutes, stirring occasionally

Beat:
  2 egg yolks until light
Add:
  ¼ cup milk
Add egg mixture to sauce
Cook 5 minutes

Combine with:
  12 oz. crab meat
Place in individual dishes or quart casserole
Heat thoroughly in hot oven and serve

BEEF AND GREEN BEANS
serves 4

Ingredients:
top round beef ¾ lb.   Tamari sauce 3 Tbs.
salt ½ tsp.   green beans ¾ lb.
vegetable oil 2 Tbs.

Preparation:
Marinate 2 hours:
    ¾ lb. top of the round beef, sliced paper thin
In:
    3 Tbs. Tamari sauce
    ½ tsp. salt

Cook in ½ cup water:
    ¾ lb. fresh green beans

In large skillet or wok heat:
    2 Tbs. vegetable oil
Add and sauté for 1 minute:
    marinated beef
Add and simmer 1 minute:
    beans and water they were cooked in
Mix thoroughly
Serve immediately

GREAT HAMBURGERS
serves 6-8

Ingredients:
ground chuck 1 ⅓ lb.   ground heart ⅔ lb.
sweet red peppers ⅓ cup   horse-radish 2 Tbs.
tomato sauce ½ cup   dry mustard 1 tsp.
chili powder ⅛ tsp.   onion ½ cup

Preparation:
Combine and mix well:
    1 ⅓ lb. ground chuck
    ⅔ lb. ground heart
    ⅓ cup diced sweet red peppers
    2 Tbs. horse-radish
    ½ cup tomato sauce
    1 tsp. dry mustard
    ⅛ tsp. chili powder
    ½ cup chopped onion
Shape into patties
Place on rack in shallow baking pan
Bake at 375° 30 minutes

MEAT LOAF
serves 4

Ingredients:

lean ground beef 1 ½ lb.
tomato sauce 1 8 oz can
oregano ½ tsp.
green or sweet red pepper ¼ cup
salt ½ tsp.

egg 1
basil ½ tsp.
prepared mustard 2 tsp.
onion ½ cup
Parmesan cheese ¼-½ cup

Preparation:

Combine and mix well:
  1 ½ lb. lean ground beef
  1 egg, beaten
  6 oz. tomato sauce
  ½ tsp. basil, crushed
  ½ tsp. oregano, crushed
  2 tsp. prepared mustard
  ¼ cup chopped green or sweet red pepper
  ½ cup chopped onion
  ½ tsp. salt
Form into loaf

Place in iron skillet or baking dish
Pour 2 oz. tomato sauce over meat loaf

Bake at 375° for 45 minutes

Sprinkle ¼ - ½ cup grated Parmesan cheese over meat loaf
Continue baking for 20 more minutes

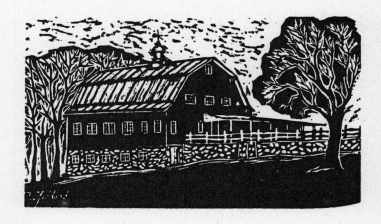

BEEF STEW
serves 6-8

Ingredients:

rump, shank or chuck beef 2 lbs.
bay leaves 2
cloves 4
onions 4
carrots 4
green pepper 1
potatoes 6 (optional)

vegetable oil 2 Tbs.
salt ¾ tsp.
allspice ½ tsp.
tomatoes 2 cups
celery ¾ cup
sweet red pepper 1

Preparation:

Heat in dutch oven:
    2 Tbs. vegetable oil
Add and brown on all sides:
    2 lbs. beef cut into 1 ½ inch pieces

Add:
    4 cups boiling water
    2 bay leaves
    ¾ tsp. salt
    4 cloves
    ½ tsp. allspice
    4 onions, quartered
Cover and simmer over low heat for 2 hours, stir occasionally

Add:
    2 cups cut tomatoes
    4 carrots, halved and cut into quarters
    ¾ cup chopped celery
    1 green pepper, cut into strips
    1 sweet red pepper, cut into strips
    6 potatoes, cut in ¼s (optional)
Cover, cook 30 minutes or until vegetables tender

Delicious on those cold winter days!

STEAK AND PEPPERS
serves 4

Ingredients:
London Broil steak 1 ½ lb.
medium onion 1
vegetable oil 2 Tbs.

large green pepper 1
mushrooms 1 cup
Ragu Italian cooking sauce 15 oz

Preparation:
Cut into ½ inch slices:
  1 ½ lbs. London Broil

Heat in skillet:
  2 Tbs. vegetable oil
Add and sauté:
  1 large green pepper, sliced
  1 medium onion, sliced
  1 cup sliced mushrooms
Add:
  1 jar (15 oz.) Ragu Italian cooking sauce
Simmer over low heat

Broil sliced steak 3 minutes on each side
Arrange steak on shallow serving plate
Pour sauce over steak
Serve immediately

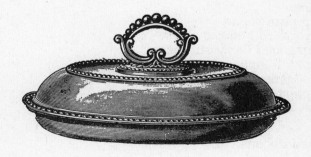

The recipes in this section are prepared with brown rice, whole grains or artichoke pasta or other starchy foods. Many LBS sufferers cannot eat these foods because they have too high a starch content. There are those who can eat a small serving while others may be able to eat a regular serving, especially if there is a good quantity of high quality protein in the same meal. So when you feel your blood sugar is under control, you may want to "take a chance" and try a small serving of these recipes.

The combination of rice or pasta and cheese or fish make a complete protein. Therefore these dishes, except Rice Plus, can be served as the main course along with vegetables.(see dialog at beginning of this section) However, you would not want to serve bread or potatoes with the meal.

NOODLES ROMANO
serves 4-6 (take a chance recipe)

Ingredients:
DeBole's whole wheat ribbons 8 oz.
Romano cheese, grated 1 cup
salt ¼ tsp. (optional)
paprika ¼ tsp.
butter 2 Tbs.

plain yogurt 1 cup
Parmesan cheese, grated ¼ cup
garlic powder ⅛ tsp.
chopped chives 2 Tbs

Preparation:
Cook according to package instructions:
    8 oz. DeBole's whole wheat ribbons

Combine:
    1 cup plain yogurt
    1 cup grated Romano cheese
    ¼ cup grated Parmesan cheese
    ¼ tsp. salt (optional)
    ⅛ tsp. garlic powder
    ¼ tsp. paprika
    2 Tbs. chopped chives

Drain:
    cooked ribbons
Stir in:
    2 Tbs. butter until melted
Add:
    yogurt cheese mixture
Heat over low heat 5-7 minutes:
    until cheese melts and mixture becomes thick
Serve immediately

SPICY LENTILS
serves 3 (take a chance recipe)

Ingredients:

clarified butter 2 Tbs.
garlic clove 1
ground cinnamon ½ tsp.
yellow lentils ½ cup
salt ¼ tsp.
shredded coconut 2 Tbs.

onion 1
green pepper 1
chili powder ½ tsp.
red lentils ½ cup
half & half 1 cup

Preparation:

Melt in large saucepan:
   2 Tbs. clarified butter
Add:
   1 sliced onion
   1 crushed garlic clove
Fry, stirring occasionally, till onion golden

Add:
   1 chopped green pepper
Fry 2 minutes, stirring frequently

Add:
   ½ tsp. ground cinnamon
   ½ tsp. chili powder
   ½ cup yellow lentils
   ½ cup red lentils
   ¼ tsp. salt
   3 cups water
Bring to boil, stirring occasionally
Reduce heat to low, simmer for 1 hour, stir occasionally

Puree mixture with handmixer or potato masher
Stir in:
   1 cup half & half
   2 Tbs. shredded coconut
Bring just to boil and then simmer 10 minutes
Serve immediately over fried rice
OR
Serve as soup with whole grain pita bread or other whole grain bread

Complete protein = lentils + milk + rice or lentils + milk + grains

Contributed by
Eswari, Roa, Luna & Chand Pattela

WHOLE CHICK-PEAS
serves 4 (take a chance recipe)

Ingredients:
dried chick peas 1 ⅓ cup
vegetable oil ¼ cup
garlic cloves 2
tumeric 1 tsp.
ground coriander 2 tsp.
large tomato 1
lemons 1 ½
cinnamon ¼ tsp.
cardamon ⅛ tsp.

salt ½ tsp.
medium onions 2
fresh ginger root 1 inch
ground cumin 1 tsp.
hot peppers 2
green pepper 1
ground cloves ¼ tsp.
allspice ¼ tsp.
parsley leaves 2 Tbs.

Preparation:
Soak overnight:
1 ⅓ cups dried chick peas
Drain and discard water

Place in saucepan:
2 ½ cups water
soaked chick peas
¼ tsp. salt
Bring to boil, cover, reduce heat to low
Simmer 1 ½ hours or till peas tender
Drain, reserve:
1 ¼ cups cooking liquid

Heat in frying pan:
¼ cup vegetable oil
Add:
2 medium sliced onions
2 chopped garlic cloves
Fry till onions golden brown, stir occasionally

Add:
1" fresh ginger root, peeled & cut in thin strips
Fry 1 minute
Stir in:
1 tsp. tumeric
1 tsp. ground cumin
2 tsp. ground coriander
Fry 5 minutes, stirring constantly
Stir in spoonful of water if mixture becomes dry

Add and cook 5 minutes:
  2 hot peppers, split open
  1 large chopped tomato
  1 green pepper, cut into strips
Stir in:
  cooked chick-peas
Cook 7 minutes

Stir in:
  reserved cooking liquid
  ¼ tsp. salt
  juice from 1 ½ lemons
Bring to boil, cover, reduce heat to low
Simmer 15 minutes
Uncover, simmer 10 minutes

Pour into warm serving dish
Sprinkle with:
  ¼ tsp. ground cloves
  ¼ tsp. cinnamon
  ¼ tsp. allspice
  ⅛ tsp. cardamon
  2 Tbs. chopped parsley leaves
Serve immediately with whole grain pita bread, or rice and yogurt salad

Contributed by
Eswari, Roa, Luna & Chand Pattela

RICE PLUS
serves 3-4 (take a chance recipe)

Ingredients:
  chicken or turkey broth 1 ¾ cups   long grain brown rice 1 cup
  onion ¼ cup

Preparation:
  Bring to boil:
    1 ¾ cups chicken or turkey broth
  Add:
    1 cup long grain brown rice
    ¼ cup chopped onion
  Cover and simmer 40 - 50 minutes
Serve with a pat of butter, salt & pepper
To make a complete protein, serve with lentils or beans.

CHEESE, RICE AND VEGETABLE BAKE
serves 8 (take a chance recipe)

Ingredients:

sunflower oil 2 Tbs.
celery 4 stalks
fresh spinach ½ cup
paprika 2 tsp.
pepper ¼ tsp.
cooked brown rice 3 cups

onions 2
mushrooms ¾ lb.
garlic clove 1
salt ½ tsp.
ground ginger ¼ tsp.
jarlsberg cheese 1 lb.

Preparation:

Heat in large skillet:
  2 Tbs. sunflower oil
Add and sauté:
  2 onions, sliced
  4 stalks celery, chopped
  ¾ lb. mushrooms, sliced
  ½ cup fresh spinach, chopped
Add and stir together:
  1 garlic clove, minced
  2 tsp. paprika
  ½ tsp. salt
  ¼ tsp. pepper
  ¼ tsp. ground ginger

Have ready:
  3 cups cooked brown rice
  1 lb. grated jarlsberg cheese

In a shallow casserole, place layers of:
  ½ the rice
  ½ the vegetables
  ½ the cheese
Repeat the layers

If food appears dry, sprinkle with a small amount of water before
  adding last layer of cheese

Bake 25 minutes at 350°

TUNA AND RICE CASSEROLE
Serves 6 (take a chance recipe)

Ingredients:

chicken broth 2 cups
butter 2 Tbs.
pepper
onion ¼ cup
tuna 14 oz.
cheddar or swiss cheese (optional)

long grain brown rice ⅔ cup
sifted oat flour 2 Tbs.
celery ½ cup
french style green beans 20 oz.
mushrooms ½ cup

Preparation:

Bring to boil:
    1 cup chicken broth or water
Add:
    ⅔ cup long grain brown rice
Cover and cook 40 - 50 minutes over low heat

In 3 quart pan, melt:
    2 Tbs. butter
Stir in:
    2 Tbs. sifted oat flour
    dash pepper
Gradually stir in:
    1 cup chicken broth
Cook and stir constantly until thickened

Stir in:
    ½ cup chopped celery
    ¼ cup chopped onion
    2 10 oz. packages frozen french style green beans (thawed)
    cooked rice
    2 7oz. cans tuna, drained and flaked
    ½ cup sliced mushrooms
Pour mixture into casserole
Sprinkle with cheddar or swiss cheese - optional

Cover, bake for 30 minutes at 350°

If desire, make ahead of time and refrigerate until about 1 hour
    before serving.
Then bake covered for about 40 - 45 minutes.

RICE CASSEROLE
serves 6 (take a chance recipe)

Ingredients:
chicken broth 1 ¾ cups
canned tomatoes 1 lb.
bay leaf 1
paprika 1 ½ tsp.

long grain brown rice 1 cup
onions 1 Tbs.
whole clove 3
cheddar cheese 1 cup

Preparation:
Bring to a rolling boil:
   1 ¾ cups chicken broth or water
Slowly stir into boiling liquid:
   1 cup long grain brown rice
Cover and cook 40 - 50 minutes over low heat

Combine in sauce pan and bring to a boil:
   1 can (1 lb.) tomatoes
   1 Tbs. minced onion
   1 bay leaf
   3 whole cloves
   ½ tsp. paprika
Cover and simmer 10 minutes.

Remove bay leaf
Pour tomato mixture into blender and blend until smooth

Spread cooked rice into greased 8" square baking dish.
Pour tomato mixture over rice
Sprinkle over top:
   1 cup grated cheddar cheese

Bake 25 minutes at 350°

CHILI RICE
serves 6 (take a chance recipe)

Ingredients:
cooked kidney or pea beans 2 cups
garlic cloves 2
green pepper 1
cooked brown rice 5 cups
chili powder 1 Tbs.

vegetable oil 2 Tbs.
large onion 1
celery stalks with leaves 2
tomatoes with juice 16 oz. can
salt 1 tsp.

Preparation:
Heat in large heavy skillet:
   2 Tbs. vegetable oil
Sauté over low heat:
   2 cloves garlic, minced
   1 large onion, chopped
   1 green pepper chopped
   2 celery stalks with leaves, chopped

Add:
   5 cups cooked brown rice
   16 oz. can of tomatoes with juice, smash up tomatoes
   2 cups kidney or pea beans
   1 Tbs. chili powder
   1 tsp. salt
Cover and heat till hot through

Let stand for 1 hour before serving
Reheat
Serve with vegetable salad

STUFFED PEPPERS
serves 6 (take a chance recipe)

Ingredients:

large green bell peppers 6	cooked small shrimp 12 oz.
cooked brown rice 1 ½ cups	cheddar cheese 1 cup
unsweetened spaghetti sauce 1 cup	fresh mushrooms ½ cup

Preparation:
Wash and remove tops and seeds from:
   6 large green bell peppers
Combine:
   12 oz. cooked small shrimp
   1 ½ cups cooked brown rice
   1 cup shredded cheddar cheese
   1 cup unsweetened spaghetti sauce
   ½ cup sliced fresh mushrooms
Spoon mixture into the peppers
Place peppers in baking dish

Bake at 350 for 45 minutes

FRIED RICE
serves 4 (take a chance recipe)

Ingredients:
brown rice 1 cup
cardamon powder ½ tsp.
peppercorns 4
cloves 10

onions 2
cinnamon 4 pieces
vegetable oil 1 Tbs.
salt ½ tsp.

Preparation:
Heat in large saucepan:
   1 Tbs. vegetable oil
Add:
   2 finely chopped onions
Sauté

Crush and add:
   ½ tsp. cardamon powder
   4 pieces cinnamon
   4 peppercorns
   10 cloves
Sauté till golden brown

Add:
   2 ½ cups water
   ½ tsp. salt
Boil for 2 minutes

Add:
   1 cup brown rice
Cover, cook till water absorbed
Serve with spiced lentils or other dishes

Complete protein = rice + lentils

Contributed by
Eswari, Roa, Luna & Chand Pattela

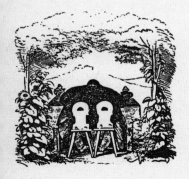

VEGETABLES

Vegetables are basically carbohydrate (starches and sugars) foods. When eating vegetables, your primary concern is what percentage carbohydrate they contain. The lower the carbohydrate content, the better it is for you when first trying to get your blood sugar stabilized The lower the percentage, the less sugar made by the body. You shouldn't eat two high percentage carbohydrates such as carrots and potatoes at the same meal. See page 180 for a list of vegetables with their percentage of carbohydrate content.

For a more complete explanation of vegetables and their percentage of carbohydrate content, see our Low Blood Sugar Handbook, particularily chapter four.

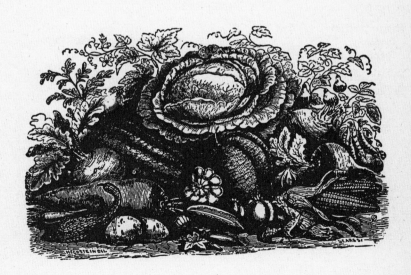

ARTICHOKES
serves 6

Ingredients:

small artichokes 6
thyme ¼ tsp.

garlic clove 1
salt ¼ tsp.

Preparation:

Trim stem of each artichoke
Remove tough leaves at base
Trim sharp tip of each leaf if desired
Put tiny pieces of garlic in each artichoke

Place in a pan of about 1 inch of boiling water:
6 small artichokes
¼ tsp. thyme
¼ tsp. salt
Cook for about 40-45 minutes, until stem is tender

Remove from water, turn upside down to drain
Serve with individual servings of a favorite dip or lemon butter

ASPARAGUS WITH CHEESE SAUCE
serves 6

Ingredients:

asparagus 1 ½ lb.
pepper ⅛ tsp.

sharp cheddar cheese 2 cups
dry mustard ⅛ tsp.

Preparation:

Steam for 10-15 minutes:
1 ½ lbs. asparagus

Melt:
2 cups sharp cheddar cheese

Add:
⅛ tsp. pepper
⅛ tsp. dry mustard
Pour melted cheese over:
steamed asparagus
Serve immediately

GREEN BEANS STEAMED
serves 3-4

Ingredients:

Green beans 1 lb.
medium onion ½

garlic powder ¼ tsp.
salt ¼ tsp.

Preparation:

Heat 1 inch of water in large saucepan
Place in steamer basket:
    1 lb. fresh or frozen green beans
Add:
    ¼ tsp. garlic powder
    ½ medium onion, sliced
    ¼ tsp. salt
Place basket of beans in boiling water
Cover, steam for about 15 minutes or until beans crunchy tender

GREEN BEANS WITH TOMATOES
serves 6

Ingredients:

olive oil 1 Tbs
medium tomatoes 4
marjoram ½ tsp.
french style green beans 20 oz.

onion ¼ cup
salt ¼ tsp.
tarragon 1 tsp.

Preparation:

Cook:
    20 oz. fresh or frozen french style green beans
Heat skillet over medium heat
Add:
    1 Tbs. olive oil
    ¼ cup chopped onion
Cook 5 minutes
Add:
    4 medium tomatoes, chopped
    ¼ tsp. salt
    ½ tsp. marjoram, crushed
    1 tsp. tarragon, crushed

Cover and simmer 10 minutes
Add:
    20 oz. cooked french style green beans
Cover, simmer until thoroughly heated

CREAMED GREEN BEANS
serves 6

Ingredients:
cooked cut green beans 20 oz.
medium onion ½
oat flour 2 Tbs.
milk 1 cup
paprika 1 tsp.

butter 2 Tbs.
mushrooms 1 cup
salt ¾ tsp.
prepared mustard 1 ¼ tsp.
almonds 2 Tbs.

Preparation:
Preheat oven to 350°
Heat 2 Tbs. butter in frying pan
Add:
   ½ medium onion, sliced
   1 cup mushrooms, sliced
Stir in:
   2 Tbs. oat flour
   ¾ tsp. salt
Gradually stir in:
   1 cup milk
   1 ¼ tsp. prepared mustard
Cook, stirring constantly until sauce is thickened
Stir cooked beans into sauce
Pour mixture into greased 1 ½ quart casserole
Sprinkle with:
   2 Tbs. sliced almonds
   1 tsp. paprika
Bake about 30 minutes or until bubbly

SPICY BEETS
serves 4-6

Ingredients:
beets 8 medium
prepared mustard 2 Tbs.
paprika ½ tsp.
pepper ⅛ tsp.

butter 2 Tbs.
worcestershire sauce 1 tsp.
salt ⅛ tsp

Preparation:
Slip into boiling water:
   8 scrubbed medium beets
Cook until tender, about 30 to 40 minutes
Hold each beet under cold running water and slip off its skin

Slice beets
Mix together and heat:
  2 Tbs. butter
  2 Tbs. prepared mustard
  1 tsp. worcestershire sauce
  ½ tsp. paprika
  ⅛ tsp. salt
  ⅛ tsp. pepper
Add:
  Sliced cooked beets
Stir together and heat
Low blood sugar sufferer, eat very small serving to see if you can tolerate beets.

PICKLED BEETS
serves 4

Ingredients:

beets 1 lb.	vinegar ¼ cup
salt ¼ tsp.	cloves 4
mustard seeds ¼ tsp.	prepared mustard 1 tsp.
dried basil ½ tsp.	pepper

Preparation:
Place scrubbed beets in pot with:
  boiling water
Cover, cook for 30-40 minutes until tender
Hold each beet under cold running water and slip off its skin

Slice beets into:
  shallow dish
Combine and pour over sliced beets:
  1 cup water
  ¼ cup vinegar
  ¼ tsp. salt
  4 cloves
  ¼ tsp. mustard seeds
  1 tsp. prepared mustard
  ½ tsp. dried basil, crushed
  dash of pepper
Chill for at least 3 hours before serving
LBS sufferer, eat very small serving to determine if you can tolerate beets.

BROCCOLI PARMESAN
serves 4-6

Ingredients:

broccoli 1 bunch
onion ½
tarragon ½ tsp.
sunflower seeds ½ cup

vegetable oil 2 Tbs.
mushrooms ½ lb.
thyme ¼ tsp.
Parmesan cheese ½ cup

Preparation:

Chop:
   stems of broccoli, break off florets
Heat in large frying pan on medium heat:
   2 Tbs. vegetable oil
Sauté:
   ½ large onion, chopped
Add and stir a minute:
   broccoli stems
Add and stir a minute:
   ½ lb mushrooms, sliced
   ½ tsp. tarragon, crushed
   ¼ tsp. thyme, crushed
   ½ cup sunflower seeds
Add:
   ¼ cup water
   broccoli florets on top
Cover, reduce heat and steam about 15 minutes

When florets are crunchy tender, sprinkle on top:
   ½ cup grated Parmesan cheese
Let cheese melt
Serve immediately and watch for finger lickin'!

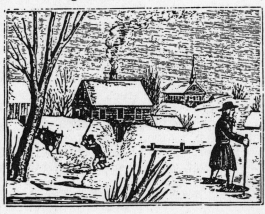

BROCCOLI
serves 4-6

Ingredients:

broccoli 1 bunch
butter 2 tsp. (optional)

lemon juice ¼ cup
salt & pepper

Preparation:

Cut broccoli into spears, if stalks thick, cut them lengthwise
Steam for about 15 minutes:
broccoli spears and leaves

Mix together and drizzle over cooked broccoli:
2 tsp. melted butter (optional)
¼ cup lemon juice
salt and pepper to taste

CABBAGE FLAIR
serves 4

Ingredients:

cabbage 3 cups
red bell pepper 1 cup
salt ¼ tsp.
pepper dash

celery 1 cup
onion ¾ cup
savory ¼ tsp.
butter 1 Tbs.

Preparation:

Heat in skillet over medium heat:
1 Tbs. butter
Combine and place in skillet:
3 cups shredded cabbage
1 cup chopped celery
1 cup chopped red bell pepper
¾ cup chopped onion
¼ tsp. salt
¼ tsp. savory
dash pepper
Stir well
Cover, cook 5 minutes stirring occasionally
Serve immediately

ORANGE, GREEN AND WHITE
serves 4

Ingredients:

vegetable oil 2 Tbs
green pepper ¼ cup
tarragon ¼ tsp.

carrots 2 cups
cauliflower 2 cups
rosemary ¼ tsp.

Preparation:
Heat in heavy skillet over med-high heat:
    2 Tbs. oil
Add, stir for 2 minutes:
    2 cups diagonally cut carrots
Add, stir 1 minute:
    ¼ cup chopped green pepper
Add, stir 2 minutes:
    2 cups chopped cauliflower
    ¼ tsp. crushed tarragon
    ¼ tsp. crushed rosemary
Stir together thoroughly
Cover and cook over low heat 10 minutes or until vegetables tender

STIR-FRIED CAULIFLOWER
serves 4

Ingredients:

safflower oil 2 tsp.
celery 1 ½ cup
red bell pepper ¾ cup
cayenne pepper dash

onion ½ cup
cauliflower 2 cups
salt ½ tsp.

Preparation:
Heat in heavy skillet over medium-high heat:
    2 tsp. safflower oil
Add one at a time, stir after each added:
    ½ cup onion, chopped
    1 ½ cups celery, chopped
    2 cups cauliflower with leaves, cut into ½ inch pieces
    ¾ cup diced red bell pepper
Stir 3-4 minutes

Add and stir well:
    ½ tsp. salt
    dash cayenne pepper
Remove from heat, let stand covered 3-4 minutes

SPROUTS (how to grow)

Ingredients:
seeds or beans (alfalfa seeds, mung beans, garbanzos, lentils etc.)

Preparation:
Place in quart or larger jar:
1 Tbs. seeds or ⅓ cup beans
Add 3 cups tepid water
Cover mouth of jar with cheesecloth, secure with rubber band
Soak overnight

Drain off all water and save to put on your plants

Rinse in tepid water and drain
Place jar on side in bag during growth
Two or three times a day for 3 to 5 days:
fill jar with tepid water
drain all water off through cheesecloth
When sprouted, place in sunlight for a few hours to green
Rinse briefly in cold water to separate sprouts
Drain in collander, store in refrigerator
Use in salads, sandwiches, soups etc.

STIR-FRIED VEGETABLES AND BEAN SPROUTS
serves 2-4

Ingredients:

vegetable oil 1 ½ Tbs.
celery ½ cup
bean sprouts ½ cup

carrots 1 cup
green peppers ½ cup
salt ¼ tsp.

Preparation:
Heat in wok or skillet:
1 ½ Tbs. vegetable oil
Add and stir for 2 minutes:
1 cup carrots, cut thin diagonally
Add and stir 2 minutes:
½ cup celery sliced diagonally
½ cup green peppers cut in strips
Add and stir 1 minute:
½ cup bean sprouts
¼ tsp. salt
Serve immediately

CHEESY EGGPLANT AND TOMATOES

serves 4

Ingredients:

vegetable oil 1 Tbs.
small onion 1
salt ½ tsp.
dried basil ½ tsp
large tomatoes 2

medium eggplant 1
green pepper ½ cup
pepper
dried oregano ¼ tsp.
Parmesan or cheddar cheese ¼ cup

Preparation:

Heat in heavy skillet:
   1 Tbs. vegetable oil
Add and sauté 4-5 minutes
   1 medium eggplant, unpeeled and diced
   1 small onion, chopped
   ½ cup chopped green pepper

Add:
   ½ tsp. salt
   dash pepper
   ½ tsp. dried basil
   ¼ tsp. dried oregano
Cover and cook 10 minutes

Add:
   2 large tomatoes, chopped
Cook uncovered 5 minutes
Stir occasionally

Sprinkle with:
   ¼ cup grated Parmesan or cheddar cheese

Smile and have your picture taken while enjoying!

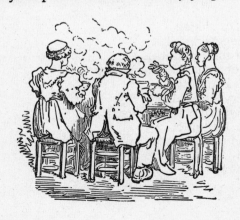

SNOWPEAS AND MUSHROOMS
serves 4

Ingredients:
vegetable oil 2 tsp.

water chestnuts ½ cup

fresh mushrooms ½ lb.

ground ginger ¼ tsp.

fresh snowpeas ½ lb.

celery 1 cup

soy sauce 1 Tbs.

Preparation:
Heat in heavy skillet over moderate to high heat:

    2 tsp. vegetable oil

Add one at a time and stir after each addition:

    ½ lb fresh snowpeas

    ½ cup sliced water chestnuts

    1 cup diagonally sliced celery

    ½ lb. fresh mushrooms, sliced

Stir-fry 2 minutes

Reduce heat to low and add:

    1 Tbs. soy sauce

    ¼ tsp. ground ginger

Let simmer 2-3 minutes

Serve immediately

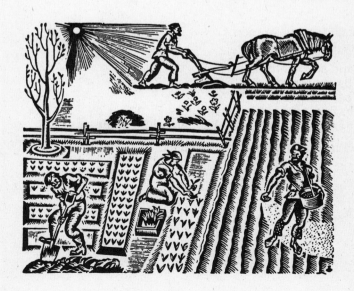

PEPPERS AND TOFU PLUS
serves 4

Ingredients:

vegetable oil 2 Tbs.
ground ginger ½ tsp.
broccoli ½ bunch
green pepper 1
soy sauce 2 Tbs.
firm tofu ½ lb.

garlic cloves 2
carrot 1
sweet red pepper 1
scallions 6
vinegar 1 Tbs.

Preparation:
Heat in skillet or wok:
    2 Tbs. vegetable oil
Add:
    2 garlic cloves, minced
    ½ tsp. ground ginger
    1 carrot, cut in ¼" slices
    ½ bunch broccoli, stems cut in thin slices, florets broken small
        pieces
Stir-fry about 2-3 minutes

Add:
    1 sweet red pepper cut in 1" pieces
    1 green pepper cut in 1" pieces
Stir-fry about 3-4 minutes

Add:
    6 scallions, cut in pieces
Stir-fry 1 minute

Add and stir gently:
    2 Tbs. soy sauce
    1 Tbs. vinegar
    ½ lb. firm tofu cut in small cubes
Cover and steam over low heat about 5-7 minutes

Enjoy with candle light and soft music

RATATOUILLE
serves 6-8

Ingredients:

vegetable oil 2 Tbs.

green pepper 1

garlic cloves 2

small fresh eggplant 1

oregano 1 tsp.

sweet red pepper 1

onions 2

medium zucchini 2

large tomatoes 2

salt ¼ tsp.

Preparation:
Heat in Dutch oven:
> 2 Tbs. oil

Add:
> 1 sweet red pepper cut in chunks
> 1 green pepper cut in chunks
> 2 onions chopped
> 2 garlic cloves minced

Sauté a couple of minutes

Add:
> 2 medium zucchini cut in 1" chunks
> 1 small eggplant cut in 1" chunks
> 2 large tomatoes cut in chunks
> 1 tsp. oregano, crushed
> ¼ tsp. salt

Cover

Steam over low heat till vegetables crisp and tender, about 15 minutes

Compliments meat loaf very nicely

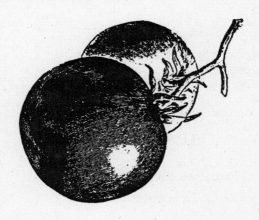

RUTABAGA AND CARROTS
serves 3-4

Ingredients:

carrots 1 cup
orange juice ½ cup
Jarlsberg cheese ⅓ cup

rutabaga 1 cup
butter 2 Tbs.

Preparation:
Mix and steam 10 minutes:
    1 cup sliced carrots
    1 cup peeled, diced rutabaga

Puree in blender till smooth:
    cooked carrots and rutabaga
    ½ cup orange juice
    2 Tbs. butter
Place mixture into buttered baking dish
Sprinkle with:
    ⅓ cup grated Jarlsberg cheese

Bake at 350° for about 30 minutes or till heated through

BAKED SPINACH
serves 4

Ingredients:

cooked chopped spinach 2 cups
eggs 2
cheddar cheese ¼ cup
Parmesan cheese ¼ cup

onion 2 Tbs.
milk ½ cup
pepper

Preparation:
Mix together:
    2 cups cooked chopped spinach
    2 Tbs. chopped onion
    2 eggs, beaten
    ½ cup milk
    ¼ cup grated cheddar cheese
    pepper to taste
Pour into greased quart baking dish

Sprinkle with:
    ¼ cup grated Parmesan cheese

Bake at 350° for about 20 minutes

SPINACH AND MUSHROOM CASSEROLE
serves 8

Ingredients:
frozen chopped spinach 30 oz.

onion ⅓ cup

butter 2 Tbs.

garlic powder dash

fresh mushrooms 1 ½ lbs.

melted butter ⅓ cup

cheddar cheese 1 ¼ cups

Preparation:
Cook and drain:

   30 oz. chopped spinach

Place in 13"x9" casserole:

   chopped spinach on bottom and part way up sides

Sprinkle with:

   ⅓ cup finely chopped onion

   ⅓ cup melted butter

   ¾ cup grated cheddar cheese

Sauté in 2 Tbs. butter:

   1 ½ lbs. fresh mushroom caps and stems

Arrange over top of cheese:

   cooked mushrooms

Add:

   dash of garlic powder

Sprinkle with:

   ½ cup grated cheddar cheese

Bake at 350° for 20 minutes or until bubbly

Contributed by
Gabriela Flannery

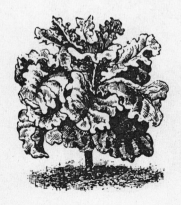

BAKED SQUASH AND APPLESAUCE
serves 3-4

Ingredients:
acorn squash 1

cinnamon

butter

unsweetened applesauce

Preparation:
Preheat oven to 350°

Wash:

    1 acorn squash

Cut squash in half and remove seeds

Place in glass baking dish:

    acorn squash, cut side down

Bake at 350° for 35 minutes

Turn squash over and bake 25 minutes more or until tender

Remove from oven

Brush inside with:

    melted butter

Sprinkle with:

    cinnamon

Fill with:

    heated, unsweetened applesauce

Eat and enjoy!

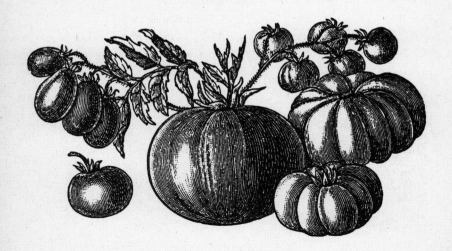

"HOT" TOMATOES
serves 4

Ingredients:
large tomatoes 2
lemon juice 1 Tbs.
paprika ¼ tsp.

horseradish 2 Tbs.
salt ¼ tsp.
parsley 1 tsp.

Preparation:
Cut in half crosswise:
  2 large tomatoes

Combine:
  2 Tbs. horseradish
  1 Tbs. lemon juice
  ¼ tsp. salt
  ¼ tsp. paprika
  1 tsp. parsley
Spread mixture over:
  tomato halves
Broil 3-5 minutes or just until heated

BAKED VEGETABLES WITH CHEESE
serves 6

Ingredients:
frozen green beans 10 oz.
mushrooms ¼ lb.
onions ¼ cup
tomato sauce 8 oz.

frozen wax beans 10 oz.
Parmesan cheese ⅓ cup
melted butter 1 Tbs.

Preparation:
Cook until thawed:
  10 oz. green beans
  10 oz. wax beans

Combine beans with:
  ¼ lb. sliced mushrooms
  ⅓ cup Parmesan cheese
  ¼ cup chopped onion
Place vegetables in 1 ½ quart baking dish
Pour over top:
  1 Tbs. melted butter
  8 oz. tomato sauce
Bake at 325° for 25 minutes

"HOT" ZUCCHINI
serves 4-6

Ingredients:

vegetable oil 2 Tbs.
carrot 1 cup
celery ¾ cup
salt ½ tsp.
dried basil ½ tsp.
tomato sauce ⅓ cup
vinegar 1 tsp.
prepared mustard 1 Tbs.

zucchini 1 lb.(4 cups)
large onion 1
medium green pepper ½
garlic powder ¼ tsp.
pepper ⅛ tsp.
chili powder ¼ tsp.
hot sauce 1 tsp
tomatoes 2

Preparation:

Heat in large skillet:
2 Tbs. vegetable oil
Add and mix together well:
1 lb. (4 cups) unpeeled thinly sliced zucchini
1 cup shredded carrot
1 large onion, chopped
¾ cup chopped celery
½ medium green pepper, cut in thin strips
½ tsp. salt
¼ tsp. garlic powder
½ tsp. dried basil, crushed
⅛ tsp. pepper
Cook covered, med.-high heat for 5 mins., stir occasionally

Combine and stir into vegetables:
⅓ cup tomato sauce
¼ tsp. chili powder
1 tsp. vinegar
1 tsp. hot sauce
1 Tbs. prepared mustard
Add:
2 tomatoes, cut in wedges

Cook uncoverd 3-5 minutes or until thoroughly heated

ZUCCHINI THAT'S CHEESY
serves 6-8

Ingredients:

butter 2 Tbs.
small onion 1
sweet red pepper ½
Parmesan cheese ⅓ cup

zucchini 4 cups
salt ¼ tsp.
celery ¼ cup

Preparation:

Place in skillet:
   2 Tbs. butter
   4 cups thinly sliced zucchini
   1 small onion, sliced
   ¼ tsp. salt
   ½ sweet red pepper, chopped
   ½ cup chopped celery
Cover and cook 1 minute over medium heat
Uncover and cook about 5 minutes, stir frequently till just tender
Sprinkle with:
   ⅓ cup grated Parmesan cheese

ZUCCHINI AND TOMATO PARMESAN
serves 4

Ingredients:

butter 1 Tbs.
onion 6 slices
dried basil ½ tsp.
pepper

zucchini 2 cups
fresh or canned tomatoes 2 cups
salt
Parmesan or cheddar cheese ½ cup

Preparation:

Heat in oven proof or stove top shallow casserole:
   1 Tbs. butter
Sauté in butter till partially cooked:
   2 cups thinly sliced zucchini
   6 thin slices of onion
Add and mix together:
   2 cups fresh or canned tomatoes, chopped
   ½ tsp. dried basil, crushed
   salt and pepper to taste
Sprinkle on top:
   ½ cup grated Parmesan or cheddar cheese
Bake at 375° for 15 minutes

ZUCCHINI HOTCAKES

serves 4

Ingredients:

zucchini 1 ½ cups
cheddar cheese ⅓ cup
mayonnaise 2 Tbs.
salt ⅛ tsp.
butter 1 Tbs.

onion 3 Tbs.
oat flour ¼ cup
oregano ¼ tsp.
pepper

Preparation:

Combine:
1 ½ cup grated unpeeled zucchini
3 Tbs. minced onion
⅓ cup grated cheddar cheese
¼ cup oat flour
2 Tbs. mayonnaise
¼ tsp. oregano
⅛ tsp. salt
dash of pepper

Melt in large skillet:
1 Tbs. butter
Spoon into skillet:
2 Tbs. zucchini batter for each cake
Flatten with spatula
Cook over medium heat, turning once till brown on both sides

Serve plain or top with:
warm tomato sauce and grated cheese
or
sour cream and chives

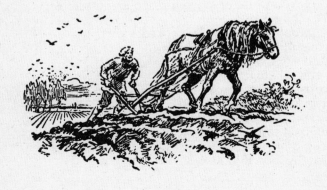

SALADS

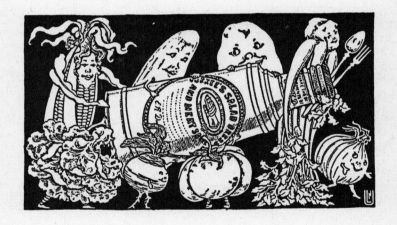

THREE BEAN SALAD
serves 6

Ingredients:

raw Scotch barley ¾ cup
bay leaf 1
navy beans ½ cup cooked
green beans 1 cup
scallions 2
fresh parsley ¼ cup
olive oil ¼ cup
basil ¾ tsp.
dill weed ¾ tsp.
pepper ¼ tsp.

soy sauce 2 Tbs.
wax beans 1 cup
cucumber 1 medium
black olives ½ cup
sweet red pepper 1
plain yogurt ½ cup
¼ cup cider vinegar
½ tsp. marjoram
¼ tsp. salt

Preparation:

Cook about 30 minutes:
    ¾ cup Scotch barley
In:
    2 cups water minus 2 Tbs.
    2 Tbs. soy sauce
    1 bay leaf
When barley cooked:
    remove bay leaf, allow to cool to room temperature

Place in large mixing bowl and mix well:
    cooled barley
    ½ cup cooked navy beans
    1 cup steamed wax beans, cut in 1 inch pieces
    1 medium cucumber, diced
    1 cup steamed green beans, cut in 1 inch pieces
    ½ cup sliced black olives
    2 scallions, minced
    1 red sweet pepper, diced
    ½ cup fresh parsley, minced
Combine and mix thoroughly:
    ½ cup plain yogurt
    ¼ cup olive oil
    ¼ cup cider vinegar
    ¾ tsp. basil
    ½ tsp. marjoram
    ¾ tsp. dill weed
    ¼ tsp. salt
    ¼ tsp. pepper
Pour liquid mixture over salad, toss until evenly coated
Refrigerate an hour then serve

CARROT SALAD
serves 4-6

Ingredients:

carrots 1 ½ lbs.
olive oil ¼ cup
fresh lemon juice 2 ½ Tbs.
parsley 6 Tbs.
dried dill 2 tsp.
pepper
sesame seeds ½ cup

cooked chick-peas 2 cups
apple cider vinegar 3 Tbs.
garlic cloves 2
scallions 4
salt ½ tsp.
cumin ½ tsp.
plain yogurt ¾ cup

Preparation:

Cut carrots into thirds, then into thin matchsticks:
   Steam till just tender

Combine in bowl:
   1 ½ lb. cooked carrots
   2 cups cooked chick-peas
   ¼ cup olive oil
   3 Tbs. apple cider vinegar
   2 Tbs. fresh lemon juice
   1 crushed garlic clove
   ¼ cup minced parsley
   4 scallions, minced
   2 tsp. dried dill, crushed
   ½ tsp. salt
   pepper to taste
   ½ tsp. ground cumin
Cover bowl tightly, refrigerate several hours

Grind in blender:
   ½ cup sesame seeds
Combine in small bowl:
   ground seeds
   ¾ cup yogurt
   2 Tbs. minced parsley
   1 ½ tsp. fresh lemon juice
   1 small garlic clove, crushed
   dash salt
Mix well
May thin to desired consistency with:
   ⅓ cup water
Chill
Serve carrot & bean mixture with spoonsful of seed & yogurt mixture
on top

RED CABBAGE SLAW
serves 8

Ingredients:
olive oil ½ cup
onion 1 Tbs.
dry mustard 1 tsp.
small head red cabbage 1
salt ¼ tsp.

lemon juice 3 Tbs.
horseradish 1 tsp.
celery seed 1 tsp.
large Granny Smith apples 3
pepper

Preparation:
Combine in large bowl:
    ½ cup olive oil
    3 Tbs. lemon juice
    1 Tbs. minced onion
    1 tsp. horseradish
    1 tsp. dry mustard
    1 tsp. celery seed
Blend well with wire whisk

Add:
    1 small shredded red cabbage
    3 large Granny Smith apples, sliced thin
Toss well

Refrigerate, covered, at least 3 hours
Stir occasionally
Add just before serving:
    ¼ tsp. salt
    pepper to taste

CAESAR SALAD
serves 8

Ingredients:
olive oil ¼ cup
hot, spicy prepared mustard 2 tsp.
fresh spinach ¾ lb.
tomatoes 3 or 4
anchovies 4

lemon juice 2 Tbs.
Worcestershire sauce 1 tsp.
bunch curly endive ½ bunch
fresh Parmesan cheese ⅓ cup
whole grain croutons 1 cup

Preparation:
Combine in small container:
   ¼ cup olive oil
   2 Tbs. lemon juice
   2 tsp. hot spicy prepared mustard
   1 tsp. Worcestershire sauce
Cover and let stand 1 hour

Wash, trim and chill:
   ¾ lb fresh spinach
   ½ bunch curly endive

Combine in large glass bowl:
   ¾ lb. spinach torn into bite size pieces
   ½ bunch curly endive
   3 or 4 tomatoes, diced
   4 anchovies, chopped
   ⅓ cup fresh Parmesan cheese, grated
   1 cup whole grain croutons
Pour dressing over salad and toss lightly
Serve immediately

COLESLAW TO YOU
serves 6

Ingredients:

medium head cabbage ½
homemade mayonnaise ⅓ cup
crushed unsweetened pineapple ½ cup, drained

celery seed 1 tsp.
unsweetened pineapple juice ¼ cup

Preparation:
Shred or chop:
   ½ medium head cabbage
Add:
   1 tsp. celery seed
   ⅓ cup homemade mayonnaise
   ¼ cup unsweetened pineapple juice
Mix thoroughly

Add and toss lightly:
   ½ cup crushed unsweetened pineapple, drained
Refrigerate until ready to serve

CUCUMBERS MARINATED
serves 4

Ingredients:
vinegar ¼ cup
salt ¼ tsp
dill weed ¼ tsp

salad oil 1 Tbs.
pepper ¼ tsp
large cucumber 1

Preparation:
Beat together:
  ¼ cup vinegar
  ¼ cup water
  1 Tbs. salad oil
  ¼ tsp. salt
  ¼ tsp. pepper
  ¼ tsp. dill weed
Add:
  1 large cucumber, thinly sliced
Toss gently
Cover and refrigerate for at least one hour

ED'S SALAD
serves 4

Ingredients:
leaf lettuce 2 cups
hard boiled eggs 3
onion ½
zucchini 1 cup
mushrooms 1 cup

avocado ½
green beans, cut 1 cup
cheddar cheese 1 cup
medium tomatoes 2

Preparation:
Combine in large bowl:
  2 cups leaf lettuce, torn into bite size pieces
  ½ avocado, diced
  3 hard boiled eggs, diced
  1 cup cooked green beans, cut
  ½ onion sliced
  1 cup cheddar cheese, cubed
  1 cup zucchini, sliced
  2 medium tomatoes, cut in bite size pieces
  1 cup mushrooms, sliced
Add:
  favorite dressing
Toss well lightly, serve immediately

PAT'S SALAD
serves 4

Ingredients:
garden lettuce 4 cups

carrots 2 cups

onion ½

cauliflower ½ cup

cooked chicken 2 cups

cucumber 1

celery 1 stalk

radishes ½ cup

Preparation:
Combine in large bowl:

4 cups garden lettuce torn into bite size pieces

2 cups chicken, cooked and diced

2 carrots, diced or shredded

1 cucumber, diced

½ onion, sliced

1 stalk celery, diced

½ cup cauliflower, diced

½ cup radishes, sliced

Add:

favorite dressing

Toss well lightly

FRESH VEGETABLE SALAD
serves 6

Ingredients:
leaf lettuce 4 cups

avocado 1

sweet red pepper 1

cucumber 1

fresh mushrooms 1 cup

cooked beets ½ cup

cooked green beans 2 cups

Preparation:
Put into large salad bowl:

4 cups leaf lettuce torn into bite size pieces

1 cup fresh mushrooms, sliced

1 avocado, diced

½ cup cooked fresh beets chopped

1 sweet red pepper diced

2 cups cooked green beans, cut

1 cucumber chopped

Pour favorite dressing over salad

Toss lightly

VENTURA'S SALAD

A salad for those desiring moments of creativity with delight tossed in.

Ingredients:

lettuce	tomato
cucumber	onion
avocado	feta cheese
black olives	oil
vinegar	salt
pepper	oregano
garlic powder	mustard
mayonnaise	

Preparation:

Combine to individual taste and desire
  lettuce
  tomato, chopped
  cucumber, sliced
  onion, sliced thinly
  avocado, chopped

Combine to individual taste:
  oil
  vinegar
  salt
  pepper
  oregano
  garlic powder
  mustard
  mayonnaise
Beat well and pour over vegetable mixture

Sprinkle on top:
  feta cheese
  sliced black olives

Contributed by
Sam & Odette Ventura and family

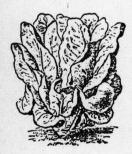

YOGURT SALAD
serves 2-4

Ingredients:
large tomatoes 2
radishes 6
young zucchini 1
salt ⅛ tsp.
paprika

cucumber ½
scallions 4
plain yogurt 1 pint
chili powder ⅛ tsp.

Preparation:
Combine in bowl, cover and chill:
   2 large tomatoes, chopped
   ½ cucumber, sliced
   6 radishes, sliced
   4 scallions, chopped
   1 young zucchini, sliced
   1 pint plain yogurt
   ⅛ tsp. salt
   ⅛ tsp. chili powder
Serve sprinkled with paprika

TUNA SALAD
serves 6

Ingredients:
mixed salad greens 3 cups
cheddar cheese 2 oz.
carrots 2
Paul Newman's Dressing ¼ cup

hard cooked eggs 2
medium tomatoes 2
tuna 7 oz.

Preparation:
Combine, cover and chill:
   3 cups mixed salad greens, torn into pieces
   2 hard cooked eggs, cut into wedges
   2 ounces cheddar cheese, cut into strips
   2 medium tomatoes, cut into wedges
   2 carrots, sliced
   7 oz. tuna, drained and flaked
Pour over salad:
   ¼ cup Paul Newman's salad dressing
Toss

Contributed by
Gabriela Flannery

EGG SALAD
serves 4

Ingredients:
hard boiled eggs 4
onion ¼ cup
salt ⅛ tsp.
prepared mustard 1 tsp.

celery ½ cup
sweet red pepper 2 Tbs.
paprika ⅛ tsp.
mayonnaise 2 Tbs.

Preparation:
Dice:
4 hard boiled eggs
Add:
½ cup celery, diced
¼ cup onion, diced
2 Tbs sweet red pepper, diced very fine
⅛ tsp. salt
⅛ tsp. paprika

Mix together and add to above:
1 tsp. prepared mustard
2 Tbs. mayonnaise
Serve on lettuce with wedges of tomato and whole grain roll

FRUIT SALAD
serves 4

Ingredients:
avocados 2
oranges 2
apple 1
cottage cheese 12 oz.

pineapple chunks in own juice 20 oz.
banana 1 (optional)
bib lettuce

Preparation:
Combine:
1 20 oz. can of pineapple chunks in own juice
2 avocados cut in chunks
2 oranges, peeled and cut in pieces
1 banana, sliced (optional)
1 apple finely chopped
Place on four plates:
nest of bib lettuce
small ball of cottage cheese in center of lettuce
fruit around cheese
Serve with whole grain muffin and butter

CREAMY MAIN DISH SALAD
serves 6

Ingredients:

unflavored gelatin 2 envelopes
mayonnaise 1 ½ cups
lemon juice ⅓ cup
salt ½ tsp.
celery ½ cup
*frozen

*concentrated pineapple juice 4 Tbs.
onion 2 Tbs.
dry mustard 1 ¼ tsp.
cooked chicken or seafood 2 cups
sweet red pepper ½ cup

Preparation:

Place in large bowl:
  2 envelopes unflavored gelatin
Add:
  2 cups boiling water
Stir until gelatin completely dissolved

Blend in with wire whisk or beater:
  4 Tbs. concentrated pineapple juice
  1 ½ cup mayonnaise
  2 Tbs. minced onion
  ⅓ cup lemon juice
  1 ¼ tsp. dry mustard
  ½ tsp. salt
Chill till partially set

Fold in:
  2 cups chopped cooked chicken or seafood
  ½ cup chopped celery
  ½ cup chopped sweet red pepper

Turn into 9"x5"x3" glass dish
Chill till firm

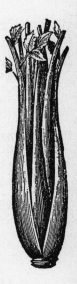

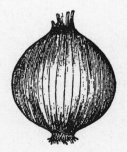

CRANBERRY SALAD
serves 8

Ingredients:

unflavored gelatin 1 envelope
cranberries 2 cups
apple 1
fresh lemon juice 2 Tbs.

unsweetened apple juice 1 ½ cups
1 tsp. orange rind
celery ½ cup

Preparation:

Pour into small saucepan:
    ¼ cup unsweetened apple juice
Sprinkle on juice:
    1 envelope unflavored gelatin
Heat over medium heat, stirring till gelatin dissolves, about
    3 minutes

Add:
    1 ¼ cups unsweetened apple juice
    2 cups chopped cranberries
    1 tsp. orange rind
    1 chopped apple
    ½ cup chopped celery
    2 Tbs. fresh lemon juice

Pour into mold
Chill until firm
Serve with turkey or chicken

CRAN-CHEESE SALAD
serves 8

Ingredients:

unflavored gelatin 2 Tbs.
fresh lemon juice ¼ cup
celery ½ cup
unsw. crushed pineapple ⅔ cups

unsw. apple cranberry juice 2 cups
cream cheese 3 oz.
walnuts ¼ cup
heavy whipping cream ½ cup

Preparation:

Pour into small saucepan:
    ¼ cup unsweetened apple cranberry juice
Sprinkle on juice:
    2 Tbs. unflavored gelatin
Heat over medium heat, stirring until gelatin dissolves, about
    3 minutes

Add to:
   1 ¾ cups unsweetened apple cranberry juice
   ¼ cup fresh lemon juice
Chill until partially set

Blend into partially set gelatin:
   3 oz. softened cream cheese
Add:
   ½ cup chopped celery
   ¼ cup chopped walnuts
   ⅔ cup unsweetened crushed pineapple, drained

Fold in:
   ½ cup heavy cream, whipped
Pour into large single mold or individual molds
Chill until set

PINEAPPLE CHEESE SALAD
serves 6

Ingredients:

unsw. crushed pineapple 9 oz. can
unsweetened pineapple jc. ¾ cup
heavy whipping cream 1 cup

unflavored gelatin 1 envelope
sharp cheddar cheese 1 cup

Preparation:
Drain:
   1 9 oz. can unsweetened crushed pineapple, save juice
Pour into small saucepan:
   ¼ cup drained juice
Sprinkle onto juice:
   1 envelope unflavored gelatin
Heat over medium heat stirring until gelatin dissolved, about
   3 minutes
Add above to:
   ¾ cup unsweetened pineapple juice
Chill until partially set
Add:
   drained crushed pineapple
   1 cup sharp cheddar cheese, shredded
Fold in:
   1 cup heavy cream, whipped
Pour into quart mold
Chill until set

SUNSHINE SALAD
serves 6

Ingredients:
unflavored gelatin 2 envelopes
lemon juice ¼ cup
carrot 1 ½ cups

orange juice 1 ¾ cups
*concentrated pineapple juice 2 Tbs.
crushed pineapple in own juice 8 oz.

*frozen

Preparation:
Pour into 5 cup blender:
    ½ cup cold orange juice
Sprinkle on juice and let stand 3-4 minutes:
    2 envelopes unflavored gelatin
Add:
    1 ¼ cups hot orange juice
Blend at low speed for about 2 minutes

Add and blend at high speed till blended:
    2 Tbs. concentrated pineapple juice
    ¼ cup lemon juice

Add and chop in blender:
    1 ½ cups carrot pieces

Pour into 8″ square glass dish

Stir in:
    8 oz. crushed pineapple in own juice
Chill till firm

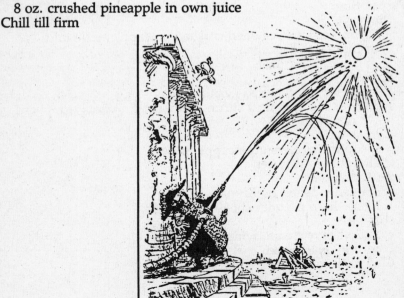

TUNA SALAD MOLD
serves 6

Ingredients:
unflavored gelatin 1 envelope
mayonnaise ¾ cup
small green pepper 1
pimiento 2 Tbs.

unsweetened Italian dressing ¼ cup
tuna fish 7 oz.
onion ¼ cup
dill weed ⅛ tsp.

Preparation:
Place in bowl:
   ¼ cup cold water
Sprinkle on top:
   1 envelope unflavored gelatin
Add:
   ½ cup boiling water
Stir until gelatin dissolved

Blend in with wire whisk or beater:
   ¼ cup unsweetened Italian dressing
   ¾ cup mayonnaise
Stir in:
   7 oz. flaked tuna fish
   1 small green pepper, chopped
   ¼ cup chopped onion
   2 Tbs. chopped pimiento
   ⅛ tsp. dill weed

Pour into:
   3 cup mold
   or
   6 individual molds
Chill till firm

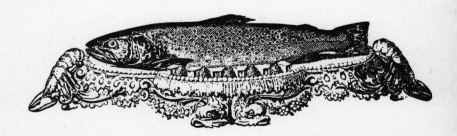

NOTES

DRESSINGS, SAUCES AND DIPS

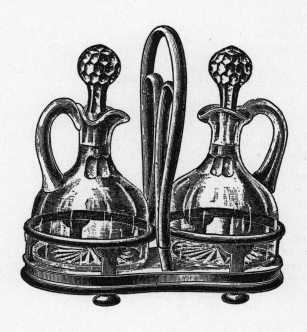

FRENCH DRESSING
makes 1 ⅓ cups

Ingredients:
vegetable oil 1 cup
salt ½ tsp
cayenne dash
paprika ½ tsp.

white vinegar ⅓ cup
dry mustard 1 tsp
onion 1 tsp.

Preparation:
Put in jar with tight lid:
  1 cup vegetable oil
  ⅓ cup white vinegar
  ½ tsp. salt
  1 tsp. grated onion
  dash cayenne
  ½ tsp. paprika
Put lid on tightly

Shake until ingredients well mixed
Store in refrigerator, shake before using

ITALIAN DRESSING
makes 1 ⅓ cups

Ingredients:
olive oil 1 cup
dried oregano ¼ tsp.
pepper pinch

vinegar ⅓ cup
dried basil ¼ tsp.
salt ⅛ tsp.

Preparation:
Combine in jar with tight lid:
  1 cup olive oil
  ⅓ cup vinegar
  ¼ tsp. dried oregano, crushed
  ¼ tsp. dried basil, crushed
  pinch of pepper
  ⅛ tsp. salt
Put lid on tightly

Shake till well mixed
Refrigerate, shake before using

RUSSIAN DRESSING
makes ¾ cup

Ingredients:

mayonnaise ½ cup
green pepper 2 Tbs
horseradish 1 tsp.

seasoned tomato sauce 2 Tbs.
onion 1 Tbs.

Preparation:
Combine:
  ½ cup mayonnaise
  2 Tbs. seasoned tomato sauce
  2 Tbs. green pepper finely diced
  1 Tbs. onion finely diced
  1 tsp. horseradish
Mix well

Store in covered container in refrigerator

MAYONNAISE
makes 1 ¼ cups

Ingredients:

egg 1
dry mustard 1 tsp
salt ¾ tsp.
vegetable oil 1 cup

lemon juice 2 Tbs.
pepper ¼ tsp
vinegar 1 tsp.

Preparation:
Combine in blender:
  1 egg
  2 Tbs. lemon juice
  1 tsp. dry mustard
  ¾ tsp. salt
  ¼ tsp. pepper
  1 tsp. vinegar
Blend at high speed until mixture is thick and lemon colored

Continue blending and add in steady thin stream:
  1 cup vegetable oil
If too thick add:
  1 Tbs. warm water
Store in covered container and refrigerate

YOGURT MUSTARD SAUCE
makes about 1 cup

Ingredients:

plain yogurt 1 cup
prepared mustard 1 Tbs.
pepper, dash

onion 1 Tbs.
salt ⅛ tsp.
paprika, dash

Preparation:
Combine and heat just until hot:
1 cup plain yogurt
1 Tbs. minced onion
1 Tbs. prepared mustard
⅛ tsp. salt
dash pepper
dash paprika
Prepare about 15 minutes before serving

Pleasant when served with baked potato, green beans, cauliflower or as a dip

CHEESE SAUCE
makes 1 cup

Ingredients:

*butter 1 Tbs.
salt ⅛ tsp.
milk ½ cup
dry mustard ⅛ tsp.

*oat flour 4 tsp.
pepper dash
cheddar cheese ⅔ cup

Preparation:
Melt in 1 quart saucepan, over low heat:
*1 Tbs. butter
Stir in until smooth:
*4 tsp. oat flour
⅛ tsp. salt
dash of pepper
Gradually stir in:
½ cup milk
Cook, stirring until thickened and smooth
Stir in:
⅔ cup grated cheddar cheese
⅛ tsp. dry mustard
Cook, stirring constantly until cheese is melted
*Butter & oat flour may be omitted, the sauce will be somewhat thinner

CUCUMBER SAUCE
about 1 ¾ cups

Ingredients:
medium cucumber 1
plain yogurt ½ cup
fresh parsley 1 Tbs.

salt ¼ tsp.
mayonnaise ½ cup
dried dill 1 tsp.

Preparation:
Peel and seed cucumber, slice into colander
Sprinkle with:
   ¼ tsp. salt
Let stand for at least ½ hr.
Combine:
   ½ cup plain yogurt
   ½ cup mayonnaise
   1 Tbs. fresh parsley, chopped
   1 tsp. dried dill, crushed
Mix in:
   sliced cucumbers

Cover and refrigerate
Serve over chilled poached fish fillets or salad

WHITE SAUCE
makes about 1 cup

Ingredients:
butter 2 Tbs.
salt ¼ tsp.
paprika, dash

oat flour 2 ⅔ Tbs.
pepper, dash
milk 1 cup

Preparation:
Melt in 1 quart saucepan, over low heat:
   2 Tbs. butter
Stir in until smooth:
   2 ⅔ Tbs. oat flour
   ¼ tsp. salt
   dash of pepper
   dash of paprika

Gradually stir in:
   1 cup milk
Cook, stirring constantly until thickened and smooth
Serve over various vegetables

CRANBERRY APPLESAUCE

Ingredients:
fresh cranberries 1 cup
apple juice ¼ cup
*frozen

large tart apples 3
*concentrated apple juice ¾ cup

Preparation:
Rinse cranberries
Wash apples in vinegar water (1 Tbs. vinegar to a quart of water)
Rinse apples
Combine in saucepan:
1 cup cranberries
3 large, tart apples, cut in eighths
¼ cup apple juice
Cook till soft

Put cooked fruit through food mill

Add:
¾ cup thawed concentrated apple juice
Cool and refrigerate
Delicious served with chicken or turkey in place of cranberry sauce

GUACAMOLE
about 1 cup

Ingredients:
ripe avocado 1
onion 2 Tbs.
garlic powder, pinch
salt

small tomato 1
lemon juice 1 Tbs.
chili powder ¼ tsp.
pepper

Preparation:
Combine in blender:
1 ripe avocado, chopped
1 small tomato, peeled, seeded and chopped
2 Tbs. chopped onion
1 Tbs. lemon juice
pinch garlic powder
¼ tsp. chili powder
salt, pepper to taste
Blend till smooth
Serve as dip for fresh vegetables or cold shrimp
Prepare as close to serving time as possible

VEGETABLE DIP
makes 2 ½ cups

Ingredients:

sour cream ¼ cup

carrrot ¼ cup

parsley 2 Tbs.

plain yogurt 2 cups

radishes 6

Preparation:

Combine:

¼ cup sour cream

2 cups plain yogurt

Add:

¼ cup grated carrots

6 radishes, thinly sliced

2 Tbs. parsley

Mix well

Refrigerate

Contributed by
Gabriel Flannery

YOGURT ROQUEFORT DRESSING OR DIP
makes ¾ cup

Ingredients:

Roquefort or Bleu cheese 1 ¼ oz.

lemon juice 1 Tbs.

pepper

plain yogurt or sour cream ½ cup

salt

Preparation:

Combine and mix well:

1 ¼ oz. Roquefort or Bleu chesse, crumbled

½ cup plain yogurt or sour cream

1 Tbs. lemon juice

salt & pepper to taste

Thin as desired with:

milk or cream

Cover and refrigerate at least 4 hours

Contributed by
Arlene McGuire

NOTES

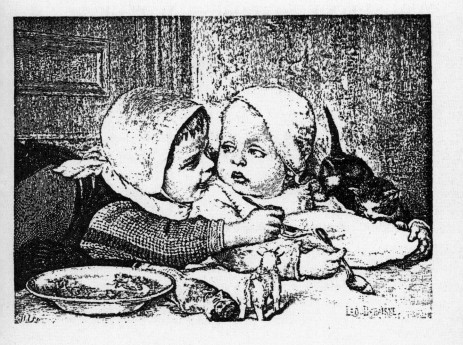

SOUPS

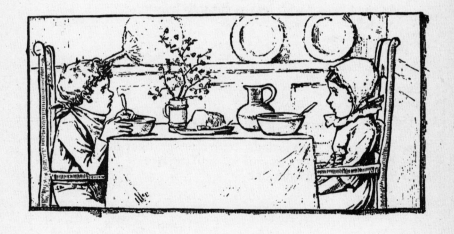

CHICKEN BROTH

Ingredients:

chicken or chicken parts 4 lbs	onion 1 large
carrot 1 large	celery stalks with leaves 2
bay leaf 1	peppercorns 6
whole cloves 4	

Preparation:

Place in soup kettle or dutch oven:
    4 lbs. chicken, whole or cut in parts
    enough cold water to cover chicken
Bring to boil
Skim off froth, if any

Add:
    1 large onion cut into eighths
    1 large carrot cut into quarters
    2 stalks of celery with leaves cut into quarters
    1 bay leaf
    6 peppercorns
    4 whole cloves
Simmer 2 hours

Cool for ½ hour
Remove chicken, strain broth

Chill broth and remove fat

Use chicken for soup, salads, casseroles or other dishes
Use broth for soup stock and for cooking rice
Broth freezes well for later use

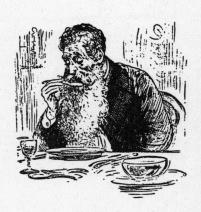

BROCCOLI SOUP
serves 8

Ingredients:

chicken broth 6 cups
onion, medium 1
sweet red pepper ¼ cup
oat flour 2 Tbs
salt ½ tsp.
milk 1 cup

vegetable oil 2 Tbs.
celery 1 cup
mushrooms 1 cup
tarragon ¼ tsp.
dill weed ¼ tsp.
broccoli 1 ½ cups

Preparation:

Heat in large saucepan or soup kettle:
   2 Tbs. vegetable oil
Add and sauté:
   1 medium onion, diced
   1 cup celery, diced
   ¼ cup sweet red pepper, chopped
   1 cup mushrooms, sliced

Stir in:
   2 Tbs. oat flour
   ¼ tsp. tarragon
   ½ tsp. salt
   ¼ tsp. dill weed

Stir while adding:
   1 cup milk
   6 cups chicken broth
   1 ½ cups broccoli
Cook until broccoli tender, stirring occasionally

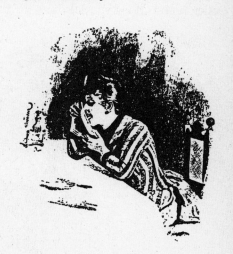

CHICKEN NOODLE SOUP
serves 4

Ingredients:

vegetable oil 1 Tbs.
onion ½ cup
tumeric ¼ tsp.
rubbed sage ¼ tsp.
salt
cooked chicken 1 cup

celery ¾ cup
chicken broth 5 cups
tarragon leaves, ¼ tsp.
cloves 2 dashes
pepper
DeBoles Substitute Fettuccine 4 oz.

Preparation:

In large saucepan or soup kettle, heat:
    1 Tbs. vegetable oil
Add and sauté:
    ¾ cup celery, diced
    ½ cup onion, diced

Add:
    5 cups chicken broth
    ¼ tsp. tumeric
    ¼ tsp. crushed tarragon leaves
    ¼ tsp. rubbed sage
    2 dashes ground cloves
    salt & pepper to taste

Bring to boil:
Add:
    4 oz. DeBoles substitute Fettuccine broken into 2 in. lengths
    1 cup cooked chicken, diced
Cook until Fettuccine tender, 8 - 10 minutes
Delicious on those special days for those special feelings!

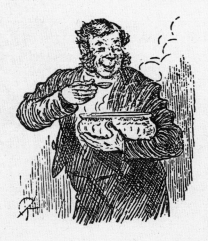

ED'S SECRET CHICKEN VEGETABLE SOUP
serves 8

Ingredients:

vegetable oil 2 Tbs.
stalks of celery 2
green beans 1 cup
green pepper ½
crushed basil ¼ tsp.
tumeric ¼ tsp.
allspice ¼ tsp.
Nature's Gourmet ½ tsp.
cooked chicken 2 cups

onion, medium 1
carrots 2
peas 1 cup
chicken broth 7 cups
sage ¼ tsp.
celery salt ½ tsp.
celery seed ½ tsp.
tomatoes 1 1lb. can

Preparation:

Heat in soup kettle:
   2 Tbs. vegetable oil
Add and sauté:
   1 medium onion, diced
   2 stalks of celery, diced
   2 carrots, diced
   1 cup cut green beans
   1 cup peas
   ½ green pepper, diced

Add:
   7 cups chicken broth
   ¼ tsp crushed basil
   ¼ tsp. sage
   ¼ tsp. tumeric
   ½ tsp. celery salt
   ¼ tsp. allspice
   ½ tsp. celery seed
   ½ tsp. Nature's Gourmet
   1 1lb. can tomatoes
Simmer until vegetables tender
Add:
   2 cups cooked cut up chicken
Simmer for 5 minutes

If a thicker consistency of soup is desired, blend:
   2 cups of soup
Return it to soup, mix together
Serve with cranberry muffins and enjoy!

MINESTRONE
serves 8

Ingredients:

chicken broth 2 quarts
large onion 1
celery 1 ½ cups
broccoli ¾ cup
green beans 1 cup
can tomatoes 1 1lb.
zucchini ½ cup
uncooked brown rice ¼ cup
dried basil 2 tsp.
salt

vegetable oil 2 Tbs.
clove of garlic 1
green pepper ½ cup
large carrot 1
fresh mushrooms ¾ cup
V-8 juice 1 cup
cooked chick peas 1 cup
dried oregano 1 tsp.
dried rosemary ½ tsp.
pepper

Preparation:

Heat in soup kettle:
   2 Tbs. vegetable oil
Add and sauté:
   1 large onion, diced
   1 clove garlic, minced
   1 ½ cup celery diced
   ½ cup green pepper, diced
   ¾ cup broccoli chopped
   1 large carrot, diced
   1 cup green beans, cut
   ¾ cup fresh mushrooms sliced

Add:
   1 1lb. can tomatoes
   1 cup V-8 juice
   ½ cup sliced zucchini
   1 cup cooked chick peas
   ¼ cup brown rice
   1 tsp. oregano
   2 tsp. basil
   ½ tsp. rosemary
   salt & pepper to taste
Simmer for about 30-45 minutes
Brings sunshine into those cold, grey days.

LENTIL SOUP
serves 4

Ingredients:
lentils 1 cup
brown rice ½ cup
basil 1 tsp.
vegetable oil 1 Tbs.
green pepper 1
celery with leaves 2 stalks
tomatoes 1 lb. fresh or canned

chicken or veg. broth or water 4 cups
salt
tarragon ½ tsp.
onion 1
carrots 2
garlic clove 1
Miso 1 Tbs. (optional)

Preparation:
Put In 2 quart saucepan:
   4 cups chicken or vegetable broth or water
   1 cup lentils
   ½ cup brown rice
   salt to taste
   1 tsp. basil, crushed
   ½ tsp. tarragon, crushed
Simmer 45 mins.

In soup pot heat:
   1 Tbs. vegetable oil
Sauté:
   1 onion, sliced
   ½ green pepper, diced
   2 carrots, diced
   2 stalks celery with leaves, diced
   1 clove garlic, minced

Add:
   1 lb. fresh or canned tomatoes
   rice and lentil mixture
   1 Tbs. miso (optional)
Simmer 15 minutes, do not boil!
Serve with green salad and whole grain bread

SPLIT PEA SOUP
serves 6

Ingredients:

vegetable oil 1 Tbs.
celery stalk with leaves 1
large carrot 1
bay leaf 1
salt ¼ tsp.
brown rice ½ cup

onion 1
green pepper ½
fresh parsley 2 sprigs
chicken or vegetable broth 5 cups
yellow split peas 1 cup
soy sauce 2 Tbs.

Preparation:

Heat in soup kettle:
　1 Tbs. vegetable oil
Add and stir a minute after each:
　1 onion, sliced
　1 stalk celery with leaves, diced
　½ green pepper, diced
　1 large carrot, diced
　2 sprigs parsley

Add:
　5 cups chicken or vegetable broth or water
　1 bay leaf
　¼ tsp. salt
　1 cup yellow split peas
　½ cup brown rice
Bring to boil
Reduce heat and simmer about 40 minutes

Add:
　2 Tbs. soy sauce
Simmer 5 more minutes
Serve with whole grain bread or muffins

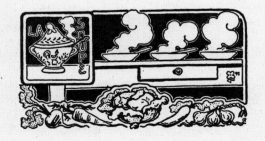

NAVY BEAN SOUP FOR SAM
makes about 9 cups

Ingredients:

dried navy beans 2 cups
vegetable oil 1 Tbs.
medium onion ½
large potato 1
white corn 10 oz.
parsley 1 Tbs.
peppercorns 7
dill weed ¼ tsp.
hot sauce 1 tsp.

large bay leaf 1
green pepper ½
celery with tops 2 stalks
carrots 2
bacon without preservatives ½ lb.
can of tomatoes 1 lb.
whole cloves 6
oregano 1 tsp.

Preparation:

Place in 5 quart dutch oven:
  2 cups navy beans, rinsed
  2 quarts of water
  1 large bay leaf
Bring to boil and simmer for 3 hours or until beans very tender

Sauté in 1 Tbs. vegetable oil:
  ½ green pepper, chopped
  ½ medium onion, sliced
  2 stalks celery with tops, chopped
Grate on large grater:
  1 large potato
  2 carrots
Add to other vegetables, cook over medium heat for several minutes
    while stirring
When beans tender, add:
  cooked vegetables
  ½ lb. bacon without preservatives, cut into bite size pieces
  10 oz. white corn
  1 Tbs. parsley
  1 1 lb. can of tomatoes
  7 peppercorns
  6 whole cloves
  ¼ tsp. dill weed, crushed
  1 tsp. oregano, crushed
  1 tsp. hot sauce
Simmer gently for about 1 hour
Stir occasionally so beans don't stick
Take out some beans and corn, put in blender and blend till smooth,
    add back to soup to make it thicker.
Add:
  salt & pepper to taste
Simmer for 15 minutes more
For fuller flavor, make a day ahead

CLAM CHOWDER
serves 4

Ingredients:
chicken broth 1 ¼ cups

small onion 1

potatoes 2 cups

salt ½ tsp.

chopped clams with juice 8 oz

butter 2 Tbs.

celery ½ cup

milk 2 cups

Preparation:
Bring to boil:
   1 ¼ cups chicken broth
Add:
   clam juice drained from 8 oz. can chopped clams
   1 small onion, sliced
   2 Tbs. butter
   2 cups diced potatoes
   ½ cup chopped celery
   ½ tsp. salt
Cover, cook until potatoes tender

Add:
   8 oz. can chopped clams
   2 cups hot milk
Heat gently, do not boil

Set aside for 1-2 hours for flavors to blend
Reheat and serve immediately

OYSTER STEW
serves 4

Ingredients:
oysters with their liquid 1 pint

salt 1 tsp.

paprika

milk 1 quart

pepper

butter 2 Tbs.

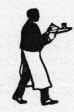

Preparation:
Scald:
1 quart of milk
Simmer for about 3 minutes over very low heat:
1 pint of oysters in their liquid until edges of oysters curl

Pour oysters into scalded milk
Add:
1 tsp. salt
dash pepper
dash paprika
2 Tbs. butter
Remove from heat, cover and let stand 15 minutes to improve flavor
Reheat just before serving, do not boil!
Stir and ladle into soup dishes

SUMMER DELIGHT
serves 2

Ingredients, chilled:
buttermilk ½ cup
avocado ½
scallion 1
carbonated water 6 ½ oz.

ripe tomatoes 2
medium cucumber 1
celery ¼ cup

Preparation:
Blend at high speed until smooth:
½ cup buttermilk
2 ripe tomatoes, peeled and quartered
½ avocado, cut in chunks
1 medium cucumber, peeled and sliced
1 scallion, peeled and chopped
¼ cup celery, strings removed and chopped

Stir in:
6 ½ oz. unsweetened carbonated water

Serve in small bowls
May top with:
fresh basil, chopped red pepper or fresh parsley

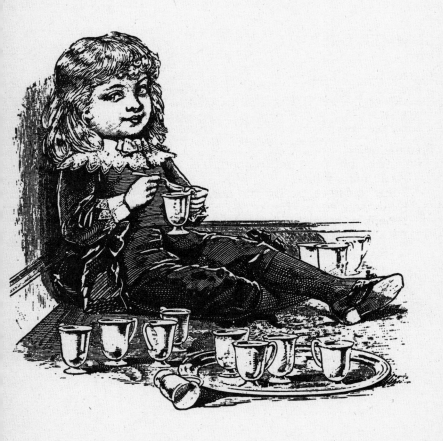

DESSERTS

The baked items are made with whole grain flours, fruits and fruit juices. No white flour, sugar, honey or artifical sweeteners are used. Fruits and fruit juices contain natural sweeteness plus vitamins, minerals and enzymes which sugar and artifical sweeteners do not contain.

The juices used are from frozen concentrates found in your local food market and liquid fruit concentrates found in health food stores.

Whole wheat pastry, oat and soy flours are the main flours used for the desserts. If using preground oat flour, rather than oat flour you have made from grinding rolled oats, be sure to sift it after measuring.

When you are just beginning to get your blood sugar stabilized, do not eat any of these desserts. After being stabilized for at least a month you may want to try a small portion. Please remember, no matter how stable you become, the key is to eat only a small serving even though it does not contain refined sugar, but fruit juices.

The gelatin desserts are made with a variety of unsweetened fruit juices and fruits to offer you some light and colorful desserts. Don't hesitate to try other unsweetened juices to add to your repertoire. Some brands of unsweetened juices are After The Fall, Apple & Eve, Dole, R. W. Knudsen, Nice & Natural, Red Cheek and Welch Orchard.

FRUITY UPSIDE-DOWN CAKE FOR...
serves 6-8

Ingredients:
apples, peaches or blueberries 3 cups
cinnamon 1 tsp.
large egg 1
whole wheat pastry flour 1 cup
baking powder 1 ½ tsp.

vegetable oil ¼ cup
nutmeg ½ tsp.
unsweetened pineapple juice ⅔ cup
oat flour ¾ cup
baking soda ½ tsp.

Preparation:
Toss together and place in 8" square baking dish:
  3 cups of slice apples, peaches or whole blueberries
  1 tsp. cinnamon
  ½ tsp. nutmeg

Beat together:
  1 large egg
  ¼ cup vegetable oil
  ⅔ cup unsweetened pineapple juice

Mix together and add to liquids:
  1 cup whole wheat pastry flour
  ¾ cup oat flour
  ½ tsp. baking soda
  1 ½ tsp. baking powder
Beat well

Pour batter over fruit
Bake at 350° for 30 minutes

Cool on rack
Turn out onto plate and enjoy!

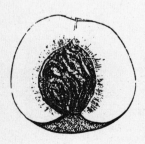
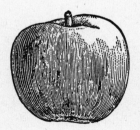

PEACH CAKE
serves 8

Ingredients:

whole wheat pastry flour 1 ½ cups
baking powder 1 tsp.
salt ¼ tsp.
eggs 2
plain yogurt ¼ cup
peaches 7
whipped cream

oat flour ¾ cup
baking soda ½ tsp.
vegetable oil ¼ cup
*concentrated pineapple juice ½ cup
vanilla 2 tsp.
sesame seeds ¼ cup

*frozen

Preparation:

Combine and set aside:
  1 ½ cups whole wheat pastry flour
  ¾ cup oat flour
  baking powder 1 tsp.
  baking soda ½ tsp.
  salt ¼ tsp.

Combine:
  ¼ cup vegetable oil
  ½ cup thawed, concentrated pineapple juice
  2 eggs, beaten
  ¼ cup plain yogurt
  2 tsp. vanilla
Add and mix well:
  flour mixture
Fold in:
  2 cups diced peaches

Pour batter into 9"x 5" loaf pan
Sprinkle with:
  ¼ cup sesame seeds

Bake at 350° for 1 hour
Serve topped with sliced peaches and whipped cream

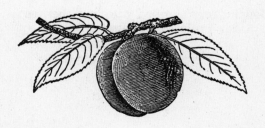

NEW YORK CHEESE CAKE
one 9" cake

Ingredients:
eggs 4
cream of tartar, pinch
plain yogurt 1 pint
nut meal or wheat germ ¼ cup
heavy cream 1 cup
cinnamon ½ tsp.

salt, pinch
ricotta cheese or cream cheese 1 lb.
vanilla 1 tsp.
lemon zest 1 Tbs.
pecans 1 cup
butter 2 Tbs.

Preparation:
Whip till stiff but not dry:
    4 egg whites
    pinch of salt
    pinch of cream of tartar

Cream:
    1 lb. ricotta cheese or cream cheese
Add and beat:
    1 pint plain yogurt
    1 tsp. vanilla
    ¼ cup nut meal or wheat germ
    4 egg yolks
    1 Tbs. lemon zest
Gently stir in:
    1 cup heavy cream
Pour mixture thru a seive
Fold in:
    egg whites

Grease a 9" springform and dust lavishly with mixture of:
    1 cup pecans, finely ground
    ½ tsp. cinnamon
    2 Tbs. melted butter (optional)

Gently pour filling onto pecan meal
Bake at 325° for 1 hour, turn off oven, leave door closed and let
    remain in oven 1 hour more

For added delight, serve topped with fresh berries
Forget basic match if calorie counting!

Contributed by
Arlene McGuire

APPLE COOKIES
about 5 dozen

Ingredients:

whole wheat pastry flour 1 cup
salt ½ tsp.
baking soda ½ tsp.
ground cloves ½ tsp.
walnuts ½ cup
vegetable oil ½ cup
rolled oats 1 cup
raisins ½ cup

oat flour ¾ cup
baking powder ¾ tsp.
cinnamon ¾ tsp.
cardamon ½ tsp.
*concentrated pineapple juice ¼ cup
eggs 2
apples 2 large
dried apricots ½ cup

*frozen

Preparation:

In small bowl, stir together:
1 cup whole wheat pastry flour
¾ cup oat flour
½ tsp. salt
¾ tsp. baking powder
½ tsp. baking soda
¾ tsp. cinnamon
½ tsp. ground cloves
½ tsp. cardamon
½ cup chopped walnuts

In large bowl, beat together:
¼ cup concentrated pineapple juice
½ cup vegetable oil
Beat in:
2 eggs
Stir in:
dry ingredients
1 cup rolled oats
2 large apples, chopped
½ cup raisins
½ cup chopped dried apricots
Mix well

Drop by teaspoon, 2″ apart onto greased cookie sheet
Bake at 350° 12-15 minutes
And hide!

APPPLESAUCE COOKIES
about 3-4 dozen

Ingredients:
*concentrated apple juice ⅓ cup
*concentrated pineapple jc. ⅓ cup
egg 1
rolled oats 3 cups
dried apricots ⅓ cup
baking powder ½ tsp.

*frozen

butter ½ cup
unsweetened applesauce 1 cup
whole wheat pastry flour 1 cup
salt ½ tsp.
baking soda ½ tsp.
cinnamon ¾ tsp.

Preparation:
Mix till light and fluffy:
⅓ cup concentrated apple juice (room temperature)
⅓ cup concentrated pineapple juice (room temperature)
½ cup softened butter

Beat in:
1 egg
1 cup unsweetened applesauce

Stir in:
3 cups rolled oats
1 cup whole wheat pastry flour
⅓ cup chopped dried apricots
½ tsp. salt
½ tsp. baking powder
½ tsp. baking soda
¾ tsp. cinnamon

Drop by tablespoon onto greased cookie sheet
Bake at 375° 12-15 minutes or until lightly browned

ALMOND BUTTER BARS
30 bars

Ingredients:
rolled oats ½ cup
almond butter about 1 ½ cups
toasted sesame seeds

wheat germ ½ cup
unsweetened toasted coconut ½ cup

Preparation:
Combine:
½ cup rolled oats
½ cup wheat germ
½ cup unsweetened toasted coconut
Add, to make a very stiff but not crumbly dough:
about 1 ½ cups almond butter
Press out with hands into a square ½ " thick
Cut into small squares
Roll in toasted sesame seeds and/or coconut
Store covered in refrigerator

Contributed by
Arlene McGuire

GRANOLA COOKIES
about 2 dozen

Ingredients:
egg 1
vanilla 1 tsp.
oat flour 1 ½ cups
baking soda ½ tsp.
walnuts ¼ cup

vegetable oil ⅓ cup
*concentrated pineapple juice ⅓ cup
salt ½ tsp.
unsweetened granola 1 ¼ cups
dried apricots ¼ cup

*frozen

Preparation:
Beat together in large bowl:
1 egg
⅓ cup vegetable oil
1 tsp. vanilla
⅓ cup concentrated pineapple juice

Mix and combine with above:
1 ½ cups oat flour
½ tsp. salt
½ tsp. baking soda

Add and mix well:
1 ¼ cups unsweetened granola
¼ cup chopped walnuts
¼ cup diced dried apricots

Drop by teaspoon onto greased cookie sheet and press lightly
Bake at 325° about 10 minutes

OATMEAL COOKIES
4 dozen

Ingredients:

dried apricots 1 cup
vegetable oil ¾ cup minus 1 Tbs.
*concentrated apple juice ⅓ cup
vanilla 1 tsp.
oat flour 2 cups
baking soda 1 tsp.
cinnamon ¾ tsp.
rolled oats 2 cups

unsweetened apple juice 1 cup
*concentrated pineapple juice ¼ cup
eggs 2
whole wheat pastry flour 1 cup
baking powder ½ tsp.
salt ¾ tsp.
cloves ¼ tsp.
sunflower seeds ½ cup

*frozen

Preparation:

Simmer for 20 minutes:
1 cup diced dried apricots
In:
1 cup unsweetened apple juice
Save:
½ cup apricot liquid

Beat in large bowl:
¾ cup minus 1 Tbs. vegetable oil
¼ cup thawed concentrated pineapple juice
⅓ cup thawed concentrated apple juice
2 eggs
1 tsp. vanilla
½ cup apricot liquid

Combine and add to above mixture:
1 cup whole wheat pastry flour
2 cups oat flour
½ tsp. baking powder
1 tsp. baking soda
¾ tsp. salt
¾ tsp. cinnamon
¼ tsp. cloves

Add:
2 cups rolled oats
apricots
½ cup sunflower seeds

Drop by teaspoon onto ungreased cookie sheet
Bake at 350° for 8-10 minutes

SPICY OATMEAL COOKIES (no flour)
4-5 dozen

Ingredients:

rolled oats 2 cups
wheat germ ½ cup
ground cloves ¼ tsp.
cinnamon 1 ½ tsp.
pecans ½ cup
vegetable oil ½ cup
*concentrated pineapple juice ¼ cup

dried milk ½ cup
salt ¼ tsp.
nutmeg ½ tsp.
unsweetened shredded coconut ½ cup
eggs 2
*concentrated apple juice ¼ cup

*frozen

Preparation:

Combine in large bowl:
   2 cups rolled oats
   ½ cup dried milk
   ½ cup wheat germ
   ¼ tsp. salt
   ¼ tsp. ground cloves
   ½ tsp. nutmeg
   1½ tsp. cinnamon
   ½ cup unsweetened shredded coconut
   ½ cup chopped pecans

Beat together and add to above:
   2 eggs
   ½ cup vegetable oil
   ¼ cup thawed concentrated apple juice
   ¼ cup thawed concentrated pineapple juice
Mix well

Drop by teaspoon onto greased cookie sheet
Bake at 300° for 20 minutes

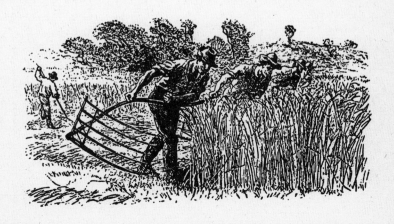

PEANUT BUTTER COOKIES
about 3 dozen

Ingredients:

butter 3 Tbs.
*concentrated apple juice ⅓ cup
unsweetened peanut butter ⅔ cup
whole wheat pastry flour 1 cup
salt ½ tsp.
baking soda ¾ tsp.

vegetable oil ¼ cup
*concentrated pineapple juice 3 Tbs.
egg 1
oat flour ¾ cup
baking powder ¾ tsp.

*frozen

Preparation:

Mix together in large bowl:
  3 Tbs. soft butter
  ¼ cup vegetable oil
  ⅓ cup thawed concentrated apple juice (room temperature)
  3 Tbs. thawed concentrated pineapple juice (room temp.)
  ⅔ cup unsweetened peanut butter
  1 egg

Combine and stir into above:
  1 cup whole wheat pastry flour
  ¾ cup oat flour
  ½ tsp. salt
  ¾ tsp. baking powder
  ¾ tsp. baking soda
Chill dough in refrigerator for about 1 hour

Roll dough into walnut size balls
Place 3 inches apart on lightly greased cookie sheet
Flatten with floured fork in crisscross design
Bake at 375° for 10 minutes, till set but not hard

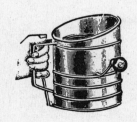

WHEAT GERM COOKIES
about 20 cookies

Ingredients:

wheat germ ¾ cup
unsweetened carob chips ½ cup
rolled oats ⅓ cup
salt ½ tsp.
egg 1
vanilla 1 tsp.

oat flour 1 cup
unsweetened coconut flakes ¼ cup
baking powder 1 ¼ tsp.
butter ½ cup
*concentrated apple grape jc. ¼ cup
*concentrated pineapple jc. ¼ cup

*frozen

Preparation:

Combine in small bowl:
   ¾ cup wheat germ
   1 cup oat flour
   ½ cup unsweetened carob chips
   ¼ cup unsweetened coconut flakes
   ⅓ cup rolled oats
   1 ¼ tsp. baking powder
   ½ tsp. salt

Cream in large bowl:
   ½ cup soft butter
   ¼ cup thawed concentrated apple grape juice (room temp.)
   ¼ cup thawed concentrated pineapple juice (room temp.)

Stir in:
   1 egg
   1 tsp. vanilla

Add dry ingredients and blend well
Place by tablespoon on greased cookie sheet

Bake at 375° for 15-17 minutes, till golden and centers firm
Cool on sheet 2-3 minutes, then remove to rack

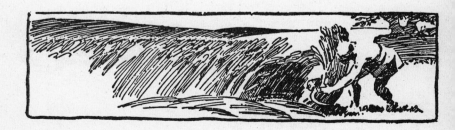

EGG CUSTARD
serves 6

Ingredients:
eggs 3
salt ⅛ tsp.
vanilla 1 tsp.

*frozen

*concentrated pineapple jc. 3 ½ Tbs.
milk 2 cups
nutmeg

Preparation:
Scald:
   2 cups milk

Beat together in medium bowl:
   3 eggs
   3 ½ Tbs. concentrated pineapple juice
   ⅛ tsp. salt
Stir in slowly:
   2 cups slightly cooled milk
   1 tsp. vanilla

Pour into six 5 oz. custard cups
Sprinkle with nutmeg

Place cups in large baking pan with 1″ hot water on bottom
Bake at 325° 40-45 minutes of till knife inserted off center
      comes out clean
Serve warm or chilled

BANANA COCONUT CUSTARD
serves 6

Ingredients:
eggs 3
milk 1 ½ cups
vanilla 1 tsp.

ripe bananas 2
nutmeg 1 tsp.
unsweetened flaked coconut 1 cup

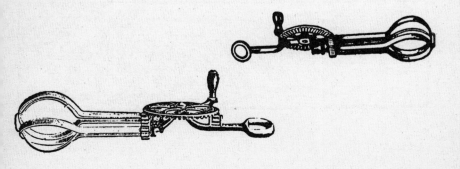

Preparation:
Blend in blender till smooth:
   3 eggs
   2 ripe bananas, sliced

Add and blend:
   1 ½ cups milk
   1 tsp. nutmeg
   1 tsp. vanilla
   1 cup unsweetened flaked coconut

Pour into eight 5 oz. custard cups
Sprinkle with:
   nutmeg if desired

Place cups in large baking pan with 1" hot water in bottom of it
Bake at 350° for 45 minutes or until knife comes out clean
Cool and refrigerate

PINEAPPLE CUSTARD
serves 6

Ingredients:

Milk 1 ½ cups	crushed pineapple in own jc. 1 ½ cups
eggs 3	vanilla 1 tsp.
ground cloves ¼ tsp.	unsweetened flaked coconut ¼ cup (opt.)

Preparation:
Blend in blender till smooth:
   1 ½ cups crushed pineapple in own juice

Add and blend together:
   1 ½ cups milk
   3 eggs
   1 tsp. vanilla
   ¼ tsp. ground cloves
Add:
   ¼ cup unsweetened flaked coconut (optional)

Pour into six 8 oz. custard cups
Set cups in large pan with 1 inch hot water in it
Bake at 350° for 45 minutes or till knife inserted off center comes
   out clean
Cool and refrigerate

APPLESAUCE

Ingredients:
tart apples-Granny Smith, Winesap
or Jonathan

Preparations:
Wash apples in vinegar water (1 Tbs. vinegar to a quart of water)
Rinse
Place in large cooking pan:
  apples cut in eighths, do not peel
Add enough water to prevent apples from sticking
Cover tightly and bring to boil

Stir occasionally, bring apples from bottom of pan to top
Cook gently till apples are soft
Put cooked apples through food mill
Let sauce cool

Pour into refrigerator containers
Refrigerate till ready to use
If desire, add cinnamon before serving
Freezes well

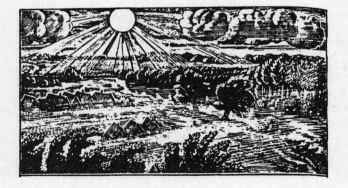

FRUIT SALAD
serves 6

Ingredients:

oranges 2
fresh blueberries ½ cup
flaked, unsweetened coconut 1 cup
orange rind 1 tsp.

pineapple chunks 1 ½ cups
fresh strawberries ½ cup
lemon juice 2 tsp.
plain yogurt 1 cup

Preparation:

Combine in bowl:
2 oranges cut in bite size pieces
1 ½ cups fresh or canned pineapple chunks, drained
½ cup fresh blueberries
½ cup fresh halved strawberries
1 cup flaked, unsweetened coconut

Combine and mix with above:
2 tsp. lemon juice
1 tsp. orange rind
1 cup plain yogurt

Cover and refrigerate at least 1 hour

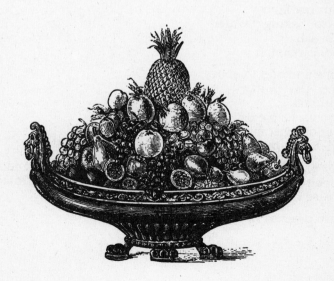

APPLE COBBLER
serves 6

Ingredients:
tart apples 6
cinnamon 2 tsp.
cloves ¼ tsp.
oat flour 2 cups
salt ¼ tsp.
eggs 2
vegetable oil ¼ cup

lemon juice 2 tsp.
nutmeg ¾ tsp.
butter 1 Tbs.
baking powder 3 ½ tsp.
cardamon ¼ tsp.
milk ½ cup

Preparation:
Slice into 8″ square baking dish:
    6 tart unpeeled apples
Pour over apples:
    2 tsp. lemon juice

Mix together and sprinkle over apples:
    2 tsp. cinnamon
    ¾ tsp. nutmeg
    ¼ tsp. cloves

Dot apples with:
    1 Tbs. butter, cut in pieces

Mix together in bowl:
    2 cups oat flour
    3 ½ tsp. baking powder
    ¼ tsp. salt
    ¼ tsp. cardamon

Combine and add to above:
    2 eggs, beaten
    ½ cup milk
    ¼ cup vegetable oil
Stir till flour just moistened
Spread dough over apples

Bake at 425° 25-35 minutes or till apples bubbly and tender and
    topping cooked underneath. If topping gets too brown, de-
    crease temperature to 375°

May use peaches in place of apples

APPLE BROWN BETTY
serves 6

Ingredients:
apples 4 cups
rolled oats ½ cup
*concentrated apple juice ⅓ cup
lemon ½

toasted wheat germ 1 cup
cinnamon 1 tsp.
butter 4 Tbs.

*frozen

Preparation:
Slice into quart baking dish:
    2 cups unpeeled apples
Sprinkle with:
    half the juice from ½ lemon

Mix together in bowl:
    1 cup toasted wheat germ
    ½ cup rolled oats
    1 tsp. cinnamon
    ⅓ cup thawed concentrated apple juice
    4 Tbs. melted butter

Sprinkle ½ oat and wheat germ mixture on top of apples

Slice into baking dish:
    2 cups more of unpeeled apples
Sprinkle with:
    remaining lemon juice
Sprinkle over apples:
    remaining oat and wheat germ mixture
Bake at 350° for 45 minutes or till apples soft and topping crunchy

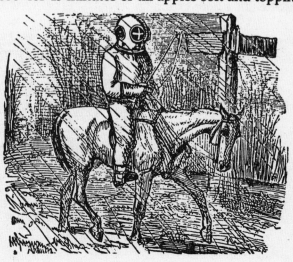

APPLE CRISP
serves 6

Ingredients:

large apples 6
cinnamon 3 ½ tsp.
*concentrated apple grape jc. 2 Tbs.
toasted wheat germ ⅓ cup
pecans ½ cup

lemon 1
allspice ½ tsp.
unsweetened granola 1 cup
butter or vegetable oil 3 Tbs.
*concentrated apple juice 2 Tbs.

*frozen

Preparation:

Slice 6 large unpeeled apples into bowl
Add and mix together:
    juice from 1 lemon
    1 ½ tsp. cinnamon
    ½ tsp. allspice
    2 Tbs. concentrated apple grape juice

Place apple mixture in:
    8″ square baking dish

Mix together:
    1 cup unsweetened granola
    ⅓ cup wheat germ
    3 Tbs. melted butter or vegetable oil
    ½ cup chopped pecans
    2 Tbs. concentrated apple juice
    2 tsp. cinnamon
Sprinkle over apples

Bake at 375° for 25-30 minutes or till apples soft & juicy
Serve warm or chilled with cream

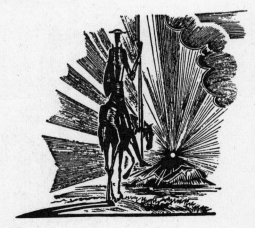

BLACKBERRY COBBLER
serves 6-8

Ingredients:
fresh blackberries 6 cups
butter 1 Tbs.
Topping as for apple cobbler (pg. 118)
*frozen

*concentrated apple juice 2 Tbs.
black cherry juice concentrate 2 Tbs.

Preparation:
Pour into 8 inch baking dish:
   6 cups fresh blackberries
Pour over berries:
   2 Tbs. thawed concentrated apple juice
   2 Tbs. black cherry juice concentrate
Dot with:
   1 Tbs. butter broken in pieces

Cover with same topping as apple cobbler
Bake at 400° 35-40 minutes
Serve warm or cold with cream

May use a combination of blackberries and sliced peaches

APPLE RASPBERRY WITH PEACHES
serves 6-8

Ingredients:
plain gelatin 2 envelopes
large peaches 2

Apple Raspberry juice 3 cups
whipped cream

Preparation:
Sprinkle:
   2 envelopes of plain gelatin
On:
   ½ cup cold water in small saucepan
Heat, stirring constantly, until gelatin dissolves completely
Add to:
   3 cups apple raspberry juice
Mix well
Place in refrigerator until slightly set
Add:
   2 sliced large peaches
Return to refrigerator until firm
Serve topped with whipped cream if desired

CHEESECAKE
serves 8

Ingredients:

unflavored gelatin 1 envelope
cream cheese 16 oz.
peaches

unsweetened pineapple juice 1 cup
vanilla 1 tsp.

Preparation:

Place in large bowl:
   1 enveloped unflavored gelatin
Add:
   1 cup scalding hot unsweetened pineapple juice
Stir until gelatin completely dissolved
Beat in with electric mixer until smooth:
   16 oz. softened cream cheese
   1 tsp. vanilla
Pour into 9 inch glass pie plate
Chill till firm
Serve topped with fresh sliced peaches or other fruit

DESSERT YOGURT GELATIN
serves 4

Ingredients:

unflavored gelatin 1 envelope
plain yogurt 1 cup
pureed peaches ½ cup
sliced peaches

orange juice 1 cup
vanilla 1 tsp.
whipped cream

Preparation:

Pour into saucepan:
   1 cup orange juice
Sprinkle on juice:
   1 envelope unflavored gelatin
Heat over low heat, stir till dissolved, pour into bowl
Chill till slightly thickened

Mix together and fold into gelatin:
   1 cup plain yogurt
   1 tsp. vanilla
   ½ cup pureed peaches

Pour into mold or individual dishes
Chill till firm
Serve topped with sliced peaches and/or whipped cream

FRESH FRUIT AND NUT GEL
serves 8

Ingredients:

unflavored gelatin 2 envelopes
plain yogurt 2 cups
almonds ½ cup
unsweetened flaked coconut ¼ cup

orange juice 1 ½ cups
crushed pineapple in own juice 8 oz.
cherries, apricots, peaches 1 ½ cups

Preparation:

Place in large bowl:
   2 envelopes unflavored gelatin
Add and stir till gelatin completely dissolved:
   1 ½ cups scalding hot orange juice

Blend in with wire whisk or beater:
   2 cups plain yogurt
Chill, stirring occasionally, till consistency of unbeaten egg

Fold in:
   8 oz. crushed pineapple in own juice
   ½ cup coarsely chopped almonds
   1 ½ cups of chopped cherries, apricots & peaches
   ¼ cup unsweetened flaked coconut
Pour into 6 cup mold or dish
Chill till firm

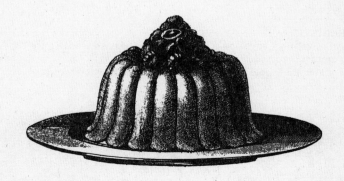

LEMON CHIFFON PIE
serves 8

Ingredients:
unflavored gelatin 1 envelope   eggs 5
lemon juice ½ cup   *concentrated pineapple jc. ½ cup
*frozen

Preparation:
Mix in medium saucepan:
    1 envelope unflavored gelatin
    ½ cup thawed concentrated pineapple juice
Blend in:
    5 beaten egg yolks
    ½ cup lemon juice
Let stand 1 minute

Stir over low heat till gelatin dissolved, about 3-5 minutes
Pour into large bowl
Chill, stirring occasionally till mixture mounds slightly when
    dropped from spoon.

Beat in medium bowl:
    5 egg whites till stiff
Fold into gelatin mixture
Turn into glass pie plate
Chill till firm
Serve topped with whipped cream if desired

ORANGE DELIGHT
serves 4-6

Ingredients:
unflavored gelatin 1 envelope   unsweetened orange juice 1 ¾ cups
heavy cream ½ cup   vanilla 1 tsp
*concentrated pineapple jc. 1 Tbs.   peaches or strawberries
*frozen

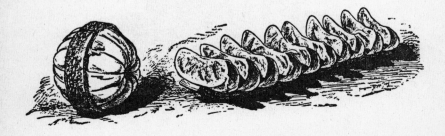

Preparation:
Pour into small saucepan:
  ¼ cup unsweetened orange juice
Sprinkle on juice:
  1 envelope unflavored gelatin
Heat over medium heat, stir constantly till gelatin dissolved
Add gelatin to and stir well:
  1 ½ cups orange juice
Cool and refrigerate till mixture becomes slightly thickened

Beat until light and fluffy:
  ½ cup heavy cream
Beat in:
  1 tsp. vanilla
  1 Tbs. concentrated pineapple juice
Blend on low speed of mixer:
  whipped cream with gelatin mixture
Spoon into dessert dishes
Refrigerate till firm
Serve topped with chilled slices of peaches or berries

ORANGE PINEAPPLE GELATIN
serves 6-8

Ingredients:

plain gelatin 2 envelopes
unsw. pineapple juice 1 ½ cups
small banana 1 (optional)

unsw. orange juice 1 ¾ cups
fresh orange 1 ½

Preparation:
Sprinkle:
  2 envelopes plain gelatin
On:
  ½ cup cold water in small saucepan
Heat, stirring constantly, until gelatin dissolved
Add to:
  1 ¾ cups unsweetened orange juice
  1 ½ cups unsweetened pineapple juice
Mix thoroughly
Place in refrigerator until slightly set
When gelatin slightly set, add:
  1 ½ orange cut in small pieces
  1 small banana, sliced (optional)
Return to refrigerator until firm

ORANGE FROZEN SOUFFLE
serves 6-8

Ingredients:
eggs 4

grated rind of 1 orange

orange juice ¼ cup

orange 1

egg yolks 3

plain gelatin 2 envelopes

heavy cream 1 ½ cups

Preparation:
Whip until very pale and thick:

4 eggs

3 egg yolks

Add:

grated rind of 1 orange

Pour into small saucepan:

¼ cup orange juice

Sprinkle on juice:

2 envelopes plain gelatin

Heat juice, stirring constantly, till gelatin completely dissolved

Add to egg mixture

Place in refrigerator

Whip till stands in peaks:

1 ½ cups heavy cream

Fold into partially set gelatin:

whipped cream

1 peeled orange cut in small pieces

Pour mixture into:

1 quart souffle dish with wax paper collar

or

a larger dish

Chill at least 4-6 hours

May be garnished with whipped cream or orange rind

Contributed by
Arlene McGuire

PEACHES AND CLOUDS
serves 6-8

Ingredients:
unflavored gelatin 2 envelopes
heavy whipping cream ½ cup
concentrated pineapple juice 2 tsp.

fresh orange juice 3 cups
vanilla 1 tsp.
peaches 4 cups

Preparation:
Pour into small saucepan:
½ cup cold water
Sprinkled with:
2 envelopes unflavored gelatin
Heat over medium heat and stir till dissolved completely

Add to:
3 cups fresh orange juice
Mix well
Refrigerate till partially set

Whip till stiff:
½ cup heavy whipping cream
Add:
1 tsp. vanilla
2 tsp. concentrated pineapple juice
Whip till mixed and peaks form
Fold into gelatin mixture

Place in 9" glass pie plate:
4 cups sliced peaches
Pour gelatin mixture over peaches
Cover and refrigerate till firm
Better if made day ahead of serving
See you in the clouds!

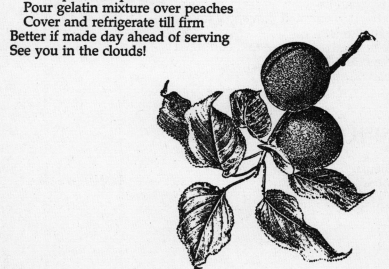

PINEAPPLE CREAM GELATIN
serves 6

Ingredients:
unsweetened pineapple jc. 3 ¼ cups
unsw. crushed pineapple 1 cup
heavy whipping cream ½ cup
*concentrated pineapple jc. 1 Tbs.

unflavored gelatin 2 envelopes
banana (optional)
vanilla ½ tsp.

*frozen

Preparation:
Pour into small saucepan:
    ½ cup unsweetened pineapple juice
Sprinkle on juice:
    2 envelopes unflavored gelatin
Heat over medium heat, stirring constantly till gelatin dissolves

Add to:
    2 ¾ cups unsweetened pineapple juice
Stir well
Cool and refrigerate till mixture slightly thickened

Add to gelatin:
    1 cup unsweetened crushed pineapple, drained
    1 thinly sliced banana (optional)
Stir well

Beat till peaks form:
    ½ cup heavy whipping cream
Add:
    ½ tsp. vanilla
    1 Tbs. concentrated pineapple juice
Fold into gelatin
Place in sherbert glasses or 5 cup mold
Refrigerate till firm
It's great!

SPANISH CREAM
serves 8

Ingredients:
unflavored gelatin 1 envelope
eggs 2
vanilla 1 tsp.

*concentrated pineapple juice ¼ cup
milk 1 ½ cups

*frozen

Preparation:
Place in medium saucepan:
  1 envelope unflavored gelatin
Beat together:
  ¼ cup concentrated pineapple juice
  2 egg yolks
  1 ½ cups milk
Stir into gelatin
Let stand 1 minute
Stir over low heat until gelatin completely dissolved, 3-5 minutes
Add:
  1 tsp. vanilla
Pour into bowl
Chill, stirring occasionally till mixture resembles egg white
  consistency
Place in bowl:
  2 egg whites
Beat till stiff
Fold into gelatin mixture
Turn into 4 cup mold or individual dessert dishes
Chill till firm

YOGURT FRUIT MOLD
serves 8

Ingredients:

unflavored gelatin 2 envelopes
orange juice 1 ½ cups
oranges 1 ½

concentrated orange juice 2 Tbs.
plain yogurt 2 cups
banana, apple, walnuts 2 cups

Preparation:
Place in large bowl:
  2 envelopes unflavored gelatin
Add:
  1 ½ cups scalding hot orange juice
Stir until gelatin completely dissolved
Beat in with wire whisk or beater:
  2 Tbs. concentrated orange juice
  2 cups plain yogurt
Chill until partially set
Stir in:
  1 ½ orange, chopped
  2 Cups, mix of sliced bananas, chopped apples & chopped
    walnuts
Pour into 6 cup mold, chill till set

NUT MEAL CRUST FOR JUST ABOUT ANYTHING

Ingredients:
butter 4 Tbs.   cinnamon ¼ tsp. (optional)
ground Brazil, hazelnuts, filberts and/or pecans 2 cups

Preparation:
Combine:
    2 cups ground nuts
    4 Tbs. melted butter
    ¼ tsp. cinnamon for dessert crust
Press mixture into pie plate

Contributed by
Arlene McGuire

OATS BRAZIL NUT PIE CRUST
8-9″ pie crust

Ingredients:
rolled oats 1 cup   Brazil nuts ¾ cup
cinnamon ½ tsp.   salt ¼ tsp.
butter ¼ cup

Preparation:
Combine in blender until finely chopped:
    1 cup rolled oats
    ¾ cups Brazil nuts
    ½ tsp. cinnamon
Pour mixture into bowl
Add:
    ¼ cup melted butter
    ¼ tsp. salt
Mix well
Press mixture onto bottom and sides of pie plate, best if use spring-
    form pan

CHEESY BANANA PIE
1 9″ pie

Ingredients:
low fat cottage cheese 1 cup   eggs 2
plain yogurt 1 cup   lemon juice 1 Tbs.
vanilla 1 ½ tsp.   *concentrated orange juice 3 Tbs.
ripe bananas 2 medium   toasted wheat germ 2 Tbs.
*frozen

Preparation:
Blend together in blender:
1 cup cottage cheese
2 eggs
1 cup plain yogurt
1 Tbs. lemon juice
1 ½ tsp. vanilla
Add, while keeping blender on low speed:
3 Tbs. concentrated orange juice
2 medium ripe bananas, sliced
Blend til smooth

Dust greased 9″ glass pie plate with:
2 Tbs. toasted wheat germ
Pour into pie plate:
banana and cheese mixture
Bake at 350° for 25-30 minutes

YOGURT PEACH PIE
1 9″ pie

Ingredients:
fresh peaches 5 cups
nutmeg ¼ tsp.
plain yogurt 1 ½ cups

cinnamon ½ tsp.
9″ nut meal crust (pg. 130)
wheat germ or nuts

Preparation:
Toss together in bowl:
5 cups sliced fresh peaches
½ tsp. cinnamon
¼ tsp. nutmeg
Pour into:
9″ nut meal crust
Top with:
1 ½ cups plain yogurt
Bake at 400° for about 25 minutes
Serve warm or cold, sprinkle with wheat germ or ground nuts

Contributed by
Arlene McGuire

YOGURT APPLE PIE
1 9" pie

Ingredients:

apples 3 ½ lbs.

plain yogurt 1 cup

9" nut meal crust 1 (page 130)

cinnamon 1 tsp.

egg 1

Preparation:

Toss together in bowl:
   3 ½ lbs. sliced, unpared apples
   1 tsp. cinnamon
Pour into:
   9" nut meal crust

Bake at 400° for 15 minutes
Remove from oven
Beat together:
   1 cup plain yogurt
   1 egg
Pour over apples

Return to oven
Bake 30 minutes more
Serve warm

Contributed by
Arlene McGuire

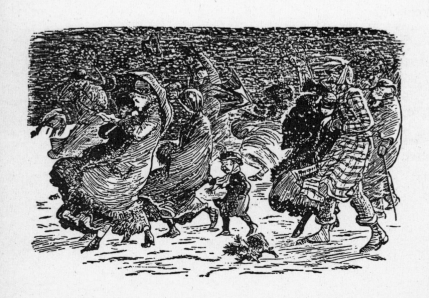

COEUR A LA CREME
serves 8-10

Ingredients:
Pot or farmer cheese 1 lb.
salt, pinch
fresh strawberries

ricotta cheese 1 lb
heavy cream 2 cups

Preparation:
Beat together till very smooth:
    1 lb. pot or farmer cheese
    1 lb. ricotta cheese
    pinch of salt

Add slowly, while beating constantly till smooth:
    2 cups heavy cream
Turn into coeur a la creme mold
If you have no mold, line a large sieve with moist cheesecloth, put weighted plate on the cheese and suspend over a bowl.

Chill overnight
Unmold
Pleasant to the eye and taste when decorated with fresh whole strawberries

Contributed by
Arlene McGuire

WHIPPED CREAM

Ingredients:
heavy whipping cream 1cup
vanilla 1 tsp.

concentrated pinapple juice 1 Tbs.

Preparation:
Chill bowl and beaters in refrigerator for at least 30 minutes
Pour into deep narrow bowl:
    1 cup heavy whipping cream
Beat on high speed till soft peaks form
Add:
    1 Tbs. concentrated pineapple juice
    1 tsp. vanilla
Beat till stiff peaks form
Refrigerate till ready to use

NOTES

SNACKS

Some of the best snacks you can have are fresh fruits and vegetables in season. Some examples are carrot and celery sticks, raw broccoli, cauliflower, green or red pepper strips and cucumbers, small servings of melons, berries, peaches, apples, pears, oranges, tangerines, pineapple, etc. Also a small handfull of nuts or some hard cheese are good to carry with you.

Keep some fresh fruits and vegetables in small handipackets in the refrigerator ready to be enjoyed or carried with you when going out.

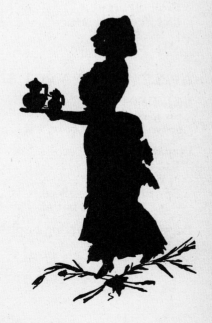

APPLE AND NUT BLOCKS
about 6 dozen

Ingredients:
unflavored gelatin 4 envelopes
heavy cream ½ cup
cinnamon ½ tsp.
apple ½ cup

apple juice 1 ½ cups
black cherry juice concentrate 2 Tbs.
vanilla ½ tsp.
walnuts ½ cup

Preparation:
Place in large bowl:
　4 envelopes of unflavored gelatin
Add:
　1 ½ cups scalding hot apple juice
Stir till gelatin completely dissolved

Stir in:
　½ cup heavy cream
　2 tbs. black cherry juice concentrate
　½ tsp. cinnamon
　½ tsp. vanilla
Chill till partially set

Fold in:
　½ cup minced apples
　½ cup finely chopped walnuts
Turn into 8" or 9" baking dish
Chill till firm
Cut into 1" squares

APPLE AND PEANUT BUTTER

Ingredients:
tart apple ½
unsweetened peanut butter 1 Tbs.

Preparation:
Cut into eights:
　½ tart apple
Spread on apple slices:
　1 Tbs. peanut butter

Eat with a small serving of plain yogurt with a dash of cinnamon

CELERY AND PEANUT BUTTER

Ingredients:
celery 1 stalk
sesame seeds ¼ tsp.

unsweetened peanut butter 1 Tbs.

Preparation:
Fill stalk of celery with:
1 Tbs. unsweetened peanut butter
Sprinkle on top:
¼ tsp. ground sesame seeds

COTTAGE CHEESE AND PINEAPPLE

Ingredients:
2% cottage cheese ½ cup
toasted wheat germ 2 tsp.

unsweetened crushed pineapple 3 Tbs.

Preparation:
Combine:
½ cup 2% cottage cheese
3 Tbs. unsweetened crushed pineapple
Sprinkle on top:
2 tsp. toasted wheat germ

COTTAGE CHEESE AND YOGURT

Ingredients:
cottage cheese ¼ cup
fruit juice concentrate (black cherry,
strawberry, etc) 1 tsp.

plain yogurt 2 Tbs.

Preparation:
Combine:
¼ cup cottage cheese
2 Tbs. plain yogurt
1 tsp. concentrated fruit juice
Experiment with different flavor concentrates or pureed fresh fruit

CRACKERS AND CHEESE

Ingredients:
cheddar cheese slices
butter ½ tsp.

Krisp & Natural Whole Wheat crackers
mustard

Preparation:
Layer on one cracker:
½ tsp. butter
slices cheddar cheese
desired amount of mustard
Place cracker on top
Serve with small piece of fresh fruit

CRACKERS AND SARDINES

Ingredients:
sardines
lettuce

whole grain crackers

Preparation:
Place on crackers:
lettuce
sardines
Limit yourself to 2 or 3 crackers and enjoy!

CHARLES' CRACKERS AND EGG

Ingredients:
Kame Cheese Rice Crackers
stuffed olives

hard boiled egg
mayonnaise

Preparation:
On each cracker place:
2 slices of hard boiled egg
tiny dap of mayonnaise
2 slices of stuffed olive
Also pleasant as a canape

CRACKERS AND PEANUT BUTTER

Ingredients:
Kavli Rye crackers 2
unsweetened peanut butter 1 Tbs.

Preparation:
Spread on cracker:
1 Tbs. unsweetened peanut butter
Place other cracker on top
Serve with:
small glass of milk
or
small dish of plain yogurt
Make up extra and store tightly wrapped in refrigerator - ideal when in a rush

STRAWBERRY YOGURT POP
makes 4

Ingredients:
plain yogurt 1 cup
fresh or frozen strawberries 10
unsweetened carbonated water 4 oz.

vanilla 1 tsp.
powdered milk 1 Tbs.

Preparation:
Blend together at high speed:
1 cup plain yogurt
1 tsp. vanilla
10 fresh or frozen strawberries
1 Tbs. powdered milk
4 oz. chilled unsweetened carbonated water

Pour into:
popsicle molds
or
4 four oz. paper cups, insert stick in center
Freeze
Enjoy!

PEACHY YOGURT

Ingredients:
plain unsweetened yogurt 1 cup   fresh peach 1
vanilla ¼ tsp.

Preparation:
Combine:
1 cup plain unsweetened yogurt
1 fresh peach, diced or pureed
vanilla ¼ tsp.
Serve with whole grain muffin
May use strawberries or other fruit in place of peaches

APPLE TASTY YOGURT

Ingredients:
Plain unsweetened yogurt ½ cup   unsweetened applesauce 3 Tbs.
cinnamon ¼ tsp.

Preparation:
Mix together:
½ cup plain unsweetened yogurt
3 Tbs. unsweetened applesauce
¼ tsp. cinnamon

ORANGE YOGURT

Ingredients:
plain yogurt 1 cup   *concentrated orange juice 1 Tbs.
vanilla ½ tsp.
*frozen

Preparation:
Combine:
1 cup plain yogurt
1 Tbs. concentrated orange juice
½ tsp vanilla

PEANUT BUTTER GRANOLA BARS
5 dozen

Ingredients:
unsweetened granola 1 ½ cups
salt ¼ tsp
toasted sunflower seeds 1 cup
toasted sesame seeds 1 cup
*frozen

dried skim milk 1 cup
*concentrated pineapple juice ⅓ cup
*concentrated apple juice 2 Tbs.
crunchy peanut butter 2-3 cups

Preparation:
Mix together:
  1 ½ cup unsweetened granola
  1 cup dried skim milk
  ¼ tsp. salt
  ⅓ cup concentrated unsweetened pineapple juice
  1 cup toasted sunflower seeds
  2 Tbs. concentrated unsweetened apple juice

Add:
  2-3 cups crunchy peanut butter, enough to make a stiff but not
    crumbly mixture

Roll mixture to a ½ inch thickness
Cut into 1 ½ inch squares
Or
Roll into small balls

Cover squares or balls with:
  1 cup toasted sesame seeds
Store in refrigerator in covered container

PEANUT BUTTER TOAST

Ingredients:
whole grain toast 1 slice
unsweetened peanut butter 1 Tbs.

butter ½ tsp.
sesame seeds ½ tsp.

Preparation:
Spread on slice of whole grain toast:
  ½ tsp. butter
  1 Tbs. unsweetened peanut butter
Sprinkle on top:
  ½ tsp. ground sesame seeds

PERSONAL PIZZA

Ingredients:
slice toasted whole grain bread 1
cheddar cheese 2 Tbs.
green pepper 2 tsp. (optional)
Parmesan cheese 1 Tbs.

Ragu Homestyle Spaghetti sauce 2-3 Tbs.
Jarlsberg cheese 2 Tbs.
mushroom 1 (optional)

Preparation:
Layer on toast:
1 ½ Tbs. Ragu Homestyle Spaghetti sauce
2 Tbs. grated cheddar cheese
1 ½ Tbs. Ragu Homestyle Spaghetti sauce
2 Tbs. grated Jarlsberg cheese
2 tsp. chopped green pepper (optional)
1 sliced mushroom (optional)
1 Tbs. grated Parmesan cheese

Place under broiler:
till cheese melts and is bubbly
Serve with vegetable salad for a small lunch

TUNA LETTUCE ROLL

Ingredients:
tuna fish
pepper

leaf lettuce

Preparation:
Place on lettuce leaf:
chunks of tuna
dash of pepper
Roll up lettuce
Savor and enjoy.

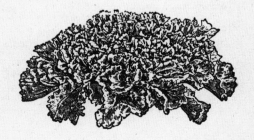

SHRIMP COCKTAIL

Ingredients:

fresh or frozen medium shrimp 4   horse-radish
unsweetened catsup

Preparation:

Mix together to desired taste:
   unsweetened catsup & horse-radish
Dip in shrimp and ENJOY!

SEASONED NUTS

makes ½ cup

Ingredients:

black walnuts ½ cup   vegetable oil ½ tsp.
salt   paprika ⅛ tsp.
cayenne ⅛ tsp.

Preparation:

Toss together:
   ½ cup walnuts
   ½ tsp. vegetable oil

Place in shallow baking pan
Roast at 300° for 15-20 minutes, till golden
Cool

Toss with:
   salt to taste
   ⅛ tsp. paprika
   ⅛ tsp. cayenne

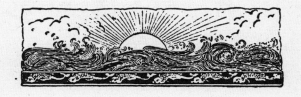

MIXED NUTS

Ingredients:

olive oil ¼ cup
soy sauce 2 tsp.
black walnuts 1 cup
peanuts 1 cup

curry powder 1 Tbs.
cayenne ⅛ tsp.
sunflower seeds 1 cup
almonds ½ cup

Preparation:

Combine in heavy skillet:
   ¼ cup olive oil
   1 Tbs. curry powder
   2 tsp. soy sauce
   ⅛ tsp. cayenne
Heat till hot

Add and stir till well coated:
   1 cup walnuts
   1 cup sunflower seeds
   1 cup peanuts
   ½ cup almonds
Place on brown paper on cookie sheet
Bake at 300° till crisp, about 10 minutes

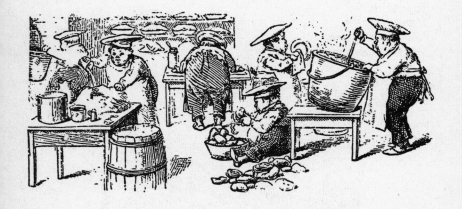

BANANA NUT DRINK
serves 2

Ingredients:

noninstant milk powder ¼ cup
unsweetened peanut butter 1 Tbs.
carob powder ¾ tsp.

small ripe banana ½
milk 8 oz.
brewer's yeast ½ tsp.

Preparation:

Blend in blender:
¼ cup noninstant milk powder
½ small ripe banana, sliced
1 Tbs. unsweetened peanut butter
8 oz. milk
¾ tsp. carob powder
½ tsp. Brewers yeast
Pour into 2 6 oz. glasses and enjoy
Drink only if you can tolerate bananas

EGGNOG
serves 1

Ingredients:

vanilla 1 tsp.
milk 1 cup
nutmeg
*frozen

*concentrated orange juice 1 Tbs.
egg 1

Preparation:

Place in blender:
1 tsp. vanilla
1 Tbs. concentrated orange juice
1 cup milk
1 egg
Blend until mixed

Pour mixture into glass
Sprinkle nutmeg on top

SHARON'S GREAT STRAWBERRY SHAKE
serves 6

Ingredients:

milk 2 cups
vanilla 1 tsp.
ice cubes 3-4

frozen unsweetened strawberries 2 cups
non-instant dry milk ½ cup

Preparation:
Blend till smooth:
    2 cups milk
    2 cups frozen unsweetened strawberries
    1 tsp. vanilla
    ½ cup non-instant dry milk
Add and blend till very cold
    3-4 cracked ice cubes
Pour into small glasses and sip slowly

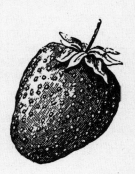

STRAWBERRY DELIGHT
serves 2

Ingredients:

plain yogurt 1 cup
fresh strawberries 10

vanilla 1 tsp.
unsweetened carbonated water 7 oz.

Preparation:
Blend together at high speed:
    1 cup plain yogurt
    1 tsp. vanilla
    10 fresh strawberries
Gently stir in:
    7 oz. chilled unsweetened carbonated water
Pour into 2 tall glasses, put feet up and relax!

STRAWBERRY COOLER
serves 1-2

Ingredients:

buttermilk 1 cup
strawberry concentrate 1 tsp. (optional)

fresh strawberries ½ cup

Preparation:
Blend together:
    1 cup buttermilk
    ½ cup fresh strawberries
    1 tsp. strawberry concentrate (optional)

ORANGE POPS OR SHAKE*

Ingredients:
plain yogurt 2 ½ cups
frozen orange juice 6 oz.

evaporated milk 13 oz.
vanilla 1 tsp.

Preparation:
Combine in large bowl:
2 ½ cups plain yogurt
13 oz. evaporated milk
6 oz. frozen orange juice
1 tsp. vanilla
Beat with electric mixer until smooth

Pour into popcicle molds
or
Pour into ten 5 oz. paper cups
Freeze 3 hours or until solid

When partly frozen insert ice cream stick in center
After frozen, put in closed container
When ready to enjoy, remove mold or paper cup
Or let stand at room temperature till soft and eat it from cup.

*Rather than freeze, drink as orange shake

YOGURT FRUIT SHAKE
serves 1

Ingredients: have all chilled
small ripe banana ¼
peach ½
plain yogurt 1 cup

strawberries 3-4
egg 1
vanilla 1 tsp.

Preparation:
Blend in Blender:
½ small ripe banana, sliced
3-4 strawberries, sliced
½ peach, sliced
1 egg
1 cup plain yogurt
1 tsp. vanilla
Pour into tall glass, sprinkle with nutmeg if desired and enjoy.

NOTES

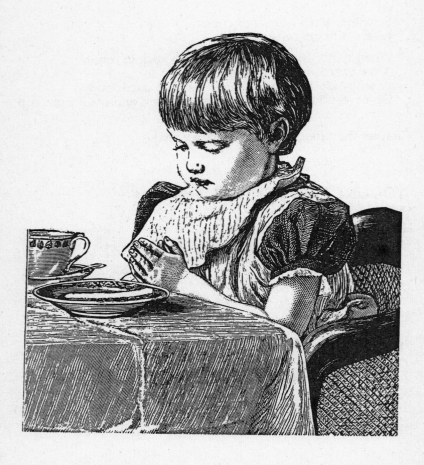

BREAKFAST

Breakfast is the most important meal of the day. It is the source of energy for getting your day off to a good start. Any wholesome food can be eaten for breakfast it doesn't have to be "traditional" breakfast food. Even something left over from dinner the night before, such as chicken, quiche, fruit salad, a whole grain muffin or yogurt. You can have a drink made from fresh fruit, milk and egg, served with a slice of whole grain bread for a great breakfast.

Forget syrup for topping whole grain pancakes and waffles. Try using fresh or frozen fruits pureed and applesause alone or mixed with plain yogurt.

If you enjoy cereal for breakfasts remember, cereals other than shredded wheat, unsweetened granola and the non instant hot cereals you prepare yourself have sugar added to them.

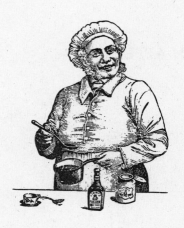

HOT BARLEY CEREAL
serves 4

Ingredients:
barley 1 cup
sesame seeds ⅓ cup
coconut ¼ cup
apple ½ cup

vegetable oil 1 Tbs
wheat germ ¼ cup
salt ⅛ tsp.

Preparation:
Grind in blender or food processor:
    1 cup pearled barley

Heat in heavy pan:
    1 Tbs. vegetable oil
Add and sauté until light brown:
    1 cup barley, ground
    ⅓ cup sesame seeds
    ¼ cup wheat germ
    ¼ cup coconut

Add:
    ⅛ tsp salt
    3 cups water
    ½ cup chopped apples

Cover and steam about 25 minutes until barley is fluffy.
Serve with milk and/or applesauce

OATMEAL WITH APPLES
serves 3

Ingredients:
rolled oats 1 cup
apple ½ cup

salt ¼ tsp.
cinnamon 1 tsp.

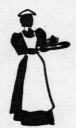

Preparation:
Pour into saucepan:
  2 cups cold water
Stir in:
  1 cup rolled oats
  ¼ tsp. salt
  ½ cup chopped apple
  1 tsp.cinnamon
Bring to boil

Cook 5 or 7 minutes, stir occasionally
Cover, remove from heat
Let stand a few minutes
Serve with small pat of butter, let melt, then add milk
Good topped with wheat germ or ground seeds

GRANOLA
serves 8-10

Ingredients:

rolled oats 2 cups
vegetable oil 2 Tbs.
sesame seeds

wheat germ ½ cup
almonds, walnuts or peanuts
sunflower seeds (unsalted)

Preparation:
Combine:
  2 cups rolled oats
  ½ cup wheat germ
  2 Tbs. vegetable oil
Spread mixture on cookie sheet
Bake 30 minutes at 250°

Mix together to make 1 cup:
  chopped almonds, walnuts or peanuts
  sesame seeds
  sunflower seeds (unsalted)
Mix nuts and seeds with baked ingredients

Bake on cookie sheet another 15 minutes

Cool, store in tight container in refrigerator
Serve ¼ cup granola topped with sliced fresh fruit and milk or plain
  yogurt.
You can use a few fingers full as an ideal snack.

BAKED EGG
serves 1

Ingredients:

egg 1   salt
butter 1 tsp.   pepper
Parmesan cheese

Preparation:
Break egg into:
   buttered custard cup
Season with:
   salt and pepper
Pour:
   melted butter over egg
Sprinkle over egg:
   Parmesan cheese
Bake at 325° about 20 minutes

EASY CHEESE OMELET
serves 1

Ingredients:

egg 1   milk 1 Tbs.
pepper   paprika
onion salt   garlic powder (optional)
cheddar cheese

Preparation:
Beat together:
   1 egg
   1 Tbs. milk
   dash of pepper
   3 dashes paprika
   dash onion salt
   dash garlic powder if desired
Pour egg mixture into:
   well buttered, heated skillet
Cook over medium heat until egg just set
Sprinkle on ½ of egg:
   grated or sliced cheddar cheese, desired amount
Turn other half of egg onto cheese
Cover skillet until cheese melts
Serve immediately with whole grain toast and butter

SCRAMBLED EGGS PLUS
serves 4-6

Ingredients:
butter 1 Tbs.
onion 2 Tbs.
green pepper 2 Tbs.
cheddar cheese ¼ cup
salt

tomato 1
mushrooms ¼ cup
eggs 6
milk 3 Tbs
pepper

Preparation:
Combine:
   6 eggs, beaten
   ¼ cup grated cheddar cheese
   3 Tbs. milk
   salt & pepper to taste

Sauté in 1 Tbs. butter in heavy skillet:
   1 tomato, chopped
   2 Tbs. chopped onion
   ¼ cup sliced mushrooms
   2 Tbs. chopped green pepper

Pour egg mixture into skillet
Cook slowly until eggs cooked, stir frequently

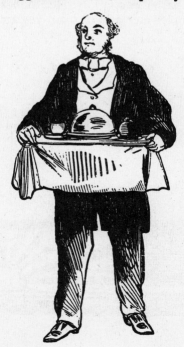

COTTAGE CHEESE PANCAKES
serves 6

Ingredients:
yogurt 1 cup
eggs 4
salt ¼ tsp.
crushed unsweetened pineapple 1 cup

cottage cheese 1 cup
oat flour 1 cup + 2 Tbs
concentrated apple juice 1 Tbs.

Preparation:
Combine in medium bowl:
　1 cup yogurt
　1 cup cottage cheese

Add:
　4 eggs
　1 cup + 2 Tbs. oat flour
　¼ tsp salt
　1 Tbs. concentrated unsweetened apple juice
Beat well, batter should be slightly lumpy

Add:
　1 cup crushed unsweetened pineapple, drained
Mix throughly

Put 1 large Tbs. of batter into lightly oiled skillet for each pancake.
Serve with butter, applesauce and/or plain yogurt.

OAT PANCAKES
serves 3-4

Ingredients:
eggs 4
milk 1 ⅔ cups
baking powder 4 tsp.
salt ¼ tsp.

vegetable oil 2 Tbs.
oat flour 2 cups
cinnamon 1 tsp.

Preparation:
Combine in medium bowl:
4 eggs beaten
2 Tbs. vegetable oil
1 ⅔ cups milk
Combine in small bowl:
2 cups oat flour
4 tsp. baking powder
1 tsp. cinnamon
¼ tsp. salt

Add dry ingredients to:
liquids
Stir thoroughly
Cook on 350 degree frying pan
Serve with applesauce or try mixture of plain yogurt & applesauce.

SOUR MILK PANCAKES
serves 4

Ingredients:

oat flour 1 ⅓ cups
baking powder 3 tsp.
salt ¼ tsp.
sour milk 2 cups

soy flour ⅔ cup
baking soda ½ tsp.
eggs 3
vegetable oil 2 Tbs.

Preparation:
Combine in small bowl:
1 ⅓ cups oat flour
⅔ cup soy flour
3 tsp. baking powder
½ tsp baking soda
¼ tsp. salt
Combine in large bowl:
3 well beaten eggs
2 cups sour milk
2 Tbs. vegetable oil

Add dry ingredients to:
liquids
Stir briskly, batter should be slightly lumpy
Cook on electric skillet at 350 - 375°
Serve with butter, unsweetened applesauce and cinnamon

WAFFLES
serves 3

Ingredients:
eggs 3
milk 1 ¼ cups
oat flour 1 ¼ cups
salt ¼ tsp.

vegetable oil 3 Tbs.
soy flour ⅓ cup
baking powder 3 tsp.

Preparation:
Combine:
  3 eggs
  3 Tbs. vegetable oil
  1 ¼ cups milk

Combine and add to above:
  ⅓ cup soy flour
  1 ¼ cups oat flour
  3 tsp. baking powder
  ¼ tsp. salt
Stir until thoroughly mixed

Pour ⅓ cup onto hot waffle grill and cook.
Serve with butter and pureed peaches or applesauce

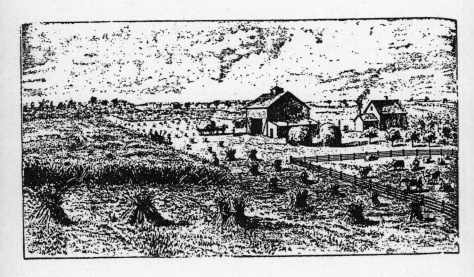

ORANGE JUICE PLUS
serves 1 (drink a breakfast)

Ingredients:

fresh orange juice 1 cup
egg 1
crushed ice ½ cup

non-instant powdered milk ¼ cup
vanilla ¼ tsp.

Preparation:
Place in blender:
1 cup fresh orange juice
¼ cup non-instant milk
1 egg
¼ tsp. vanilla
½ cup crushed ice
Blend till well blended
Serve with slice of whole grain toast

STRAWBERRY MILKSHAKE
serves 1 (drink a breakfast)

Ingredients:

fresh milk ½ cup
egg 1
non-instant powdered milk 3 Tbs.

fresh or frozen strawberries ½ cup
vanilla ½ tsp.
ice cubes 1

Preparation:
Combine in blender:
½ cup fresh milk
½ cup strawberries, fresh or frozen
1 egg
½ tsp. vanilla
3 Tbs. non-instant powdered milk
Blend till mixed

Add:
1 ice cube, cracked
Blend again
Serve with whole grain muffin or bread and butter

NOTES

BREADS

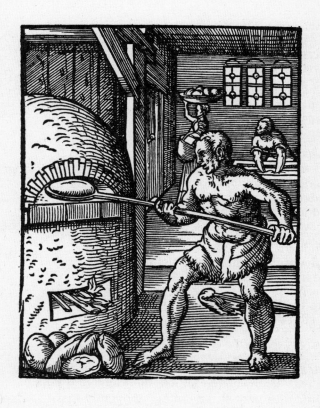

FRENCH BREAD
2 loaves

Ingredients:
yogurt 1 cup
salt 2 tsp.
oat flour 1 cup
egg white 1

active dry yeast 1 envelope
whole wheat flour 5 cups
corn meal

Preparation:
Combine:
   2 cups hot water
   1 cup yogurt
Their combined temperature should be about 105°

Add:
   1 envelope active dry yeast
When yeast dissolved, stir in:
   3 cups whole wheat flour
Beat well until dough becomes smooth

Add and mix well after each cup:
   2 Tsp. salt
   2 cups whole wheat flour, cup by cup
   1 cup oat flour

Turn dough out onto lightly floured board
Knead for about 10 minutes, or until dough is no longer sticky,
   adding additional flour until dough is stiff
Place dough in lightly greased bowl
Turn dough once to grease surface
Cover with teatowel and let rise until double in bulk, about 1 hour

Punch down
Turn dough out onto lightly floured board
Divide in half
Roll each half into 15"x8" oblong shape
Roll up tightly as for jelly roll
Pinch edges together

Grease one large or 2 small cookie sheets
Dust with cornmeal
Place loaves on cookie sheet
Cover with teatowel and let rise till doubled in bulk
If desire, with very sharp knife, very gently make ½" deep
slashes across bread 2" apart

Combine:
  1 beaten egg white
  1 Tbs. cold water
Very gently brush mixture on top of each loaf
Preheat oven to 400°
Bake about 40 minutes
Remove from cookie sheet and cool on rack

WHOLE GRAIN BREAD
2 loaves

Ingredients:

whole wheat flour 4-5 cups   active dry yeast 2 envelopes
salt 1 tsp.   triticale flour 2 cups

Preparation:
Place in large bowl and mix together:
  3 cups whole wheat flour
  2 envelopes active dry yeast
  1 tsp. salt
Gradually add:
  3 cups very warm water (120-130°)
Beat 2 minutes at medium speed, scraping bowl occasionally
Add:
  1 cup whole wheat flour
Beat 2 minutes at high speed, scraping bowl occasionally
Stir in:
  2 cups triticale flour
Sprinkle on kneading surface:
  whole wheat flour
Knead 8-10 minutes, till smooth and elastic
Cover with plastic wrap and tea towel
Let rest 20 minutes

Punch down, divide dough in half
Shape into 2 loaves
Place in 2 greased 9" × 5" × 3" bread pans
Cover with plastic wrap, place in refrigerator for 2-24 hours

When ready to bake, remove from refrigerator 10 minutes ahead
Uncover, puncture any air bubbles
Bake at 375° about 45 minutes
Remove from pans, cool on rack

PAT'S THREE GRAIN BREAD
2 loaves

Ingredients at room temperature:
whole wheat flour 5 cups
salt 2 tsp.
vegetable oil ⅓ cup
soy flour ⅓ cup
oat flour 2 ¼ cups

active dry yeast 2 envelopes
non-instant powdered milk ⅔ cup
eggs 2
triticale flour 1 cup

Preparation:
Stir together in large mixing bowl:
    3 cups whole wheat flour
    2 envelopes active dry yeast
    2 tsp. salt
    ⅔ cup powdered milk

Add:
    ⅓ cup vegetable oil
    2 eggs
    2 cups very warm water (120°)
Beat 5-10 minutes on medium speed of electric mixer
Mix together and stir in by hand:
    ⅓ cup soy flour
    1 cup triticale flour
    1 ¼ cups oat flour
Stir in:
    1 cup oat flour
    1 cup whole wheat flour
Sprinkle on kneading surface:
    1 cup whole wheat flour
Turn dough onto floured surface
Oil hands and knead 5-10 minutes till dough smooth and elastic
Add additional whole wheat flour as necessary

Cover with plastic wrap and folded tea towel
Let rest 20 minutes

Punch down by kneading a few times
Divide into 2 equal parts, shape into loaves
Place into 2 well greased 9"x5"x3" bread pans
Cover with plastic wrap and refrigerate from 2-24 hours

When ready to bake, remove from refrigerator 10 minutes ahead
Uncover and puncture any air bubbles
Bake at 350° for 35-45 minutes
Remove from pans, allow to cool on rack and enjoy!

PUMPERNICKEL BREAD
2 loaves

Ingredients:
active dry yeast 2 envelopes
rye flour 2 cups
cornmeal ⅓ cup
salt 2 tsp.

whole wheat flour 5-6 cups
buckwheat flour ⅔ cup
soy flour ⅓ cup

Preparation:
Pour into a large bowl:
 5 cups warm (105°) water
Add:
 2 Tbs. active dry yeast

When yeast dissolved, stir in:
 3 cups whole wheat flour
Beat very well

Add:
 2 cups whole wheat flour, cup by cup
Mix well after each cup

Mix together:
 2 cups rye flour
 ⅔ cup buckwheat flour
 ⅓ cup cornmeal
 ⅓ cup soy flour
 2 tsp. salt
Add cup by cup to wheat mixture
Mix well after each addition

Turn dough out onto floured board
Knead well, about 10 minutes, adding whole wheat flour as needed

Place dough in greased bowl, turning once
Cover and let rise till double in bulk, about 1 hour

Punch dough down
Turn dough out onto lightly floured board
Divide dough in half
Shape into loaves
Place in 2 9"x5"x3" loaf pans

Cover and let rise till rounded just above rim of pan, about 1 hour
Preheat oven to 375°
Bake for about 1 hour

OAT BREAD
2 loaves

Ingredients:
rolled oats 3 cups

salt 2 tsp.

whole wheat flour 4-5 cups

non-instant dried milk ½ cup

vegetable oil 2 Tbs.

active dry yeast 1 envelope

oat flour 1 ½ cups

toasted wheat germ ½ cup

Preparation:
Place in medium bowl:
>   3 cups rolled oats
>   2 Tbs. vegetable oil
>   2 tsp. salt

Pour over oats:
>   2 cups boiling water

Set aside and let cool to lukewarm

Sift together:
>   4 cups whole wheat flour
>   ½ cup non-instant dried milk

Mix together in large bowl:
>   1 ½ cups flour milk mixture
>   1 envelope active dry yeast

Add:
>   1 ½ cups warm water, 105°

Beat well until dough becomes smooth

Add and beat well after each cup:
>   2 cups flour milk mixture

Add and mix well:
>   oat mixture

Add and mix well:
>   1 ½ cups oat flour

Add and mix well:
>   ½ cup wheat germ

Turn out onto floured board

Knead in:
>   rest of flour milk mixture
>   more whole wheat flour if needed

Place in greased bowl, let rise till double in bulk

Punch down, form into two loaves

Place in two 8"x4" loaf pans, let rise till double in bulk

Bake for about 45 minutes at 400°

PARKER HOUSE ROLLS
makes 2-3 dozen rolls

Ingredients: have at room temperature

yeast 1 envelope

egg 1

whole wheat flour 3 ½-4 ½ cups

vegetable oil 2 Tbs.

salt 1 tsp.

butter

Preparation:
Stir together:
>1 ½ cups warm water 105-110°
>1 envelope yeast
>2 Tbs. vegetable oil
>1 egg
>1 tsp. salt

Gradually stir in to make soft dough:
>2-3 cups whole wheat flour

Beat vigorously

Knead in remaining flour until smooth

Place dough in oiled bowl, turn once
Cover, let rise in warm place (80-85°) until double in bulk
>about 1 hr.

Punch dough down
Turn out onto lightly floured board
Divide dough in half
Roll each half into ½" thick circle

Cut with 2 ½" biscuit cutter
Brush with very soft butter
Make crease, just off center, with back of knife
Fold larger side over smaller so edges just meet
Pinch end edges together

Place on greased cookie sheet, so rolls almost touching
Brush very lightly with melted butter or oil

Cover, let rise until double in bulk, about 1 hour
Bake at 400° about 10-15 minutes

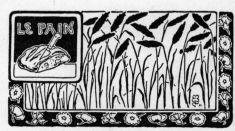

UNLEAVENED BREAD
serves 8

Ingredients:

whole wheat pastry flour 2 cups
butter 4 Tbs.

salt ½ tsp.
melted butter 1 Tbs

Preparation:

Sift together into large bowl:
  2 cups whole wheat pastry flour
  ½ tsp. salt

Add:
  4 Tbs. soft butter
Rub into flour with fingers

Make well in center of flour, pour in:
  ⅓ cup water
Gradually add, while mixing water and flour with fingers:
  ⅓ cup water
Form dough into ball

Place on floured board
Knead for about 10 minutes or till elastic
Place dough back in bowl, cover, let rest for 30 mins. at room
   temperature

Divide dough into:
  8 equal portions
Roll each portion into:
  thin, round shape, 6″ in diameter

Heat heavy skillet over moderate heat
When hot, put 1 round into pan
When small blisters appear, press to flatten dough

Turn over, cook till pale golden
Remove from pan, brush with a little melted butter
Serve and enjoy while warm

Contributed by
Eswari, Roa, Luna & Chand Pattela

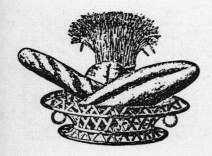

I truly enjoy muffins but I do not enjoy washing the muffin tin. So to avoid this, I now use an 8" square baking dish which is far less troublesome to wash. You must remember to allow the muffins to cook a little longer than if they were in a muffin tin. Give it a try.

APPLE MUFFINS
12 muffins

Ingredients:
oat flour ¼ cup

baking powder 4 tsp.

cinnamon ¾ tsp.

eggs 2

milk ½ cup

chopped apples 1 cup

whole wheat pastry flour 1 ¾ cups

salt ½ tsp.

nutmeg ¼ tsp.

apple juice ½ cup.

vegetable oil ¼ cup

Preparation:
Combine in medium bowl:
1 ¾ cups whole wheat pastry flour
¼ cup oat flour
4 tsp. baking powder
½ tsp. salt
¾ tsp. cinnamon
¼ tsp. nutmeg

Combine in small bowl:
2 eggs, beaten
½ cup apple juice
½ cup milk
¼ cup vegetable oil

Add liquids to:
flour mixture
Stir just till moistened

Fold in:
1 cup chopped apples

Spoon batter into greased muffin tins
Bake at 400° about 20 minutes

APPLESAUCE MUFFINS
12 muffins

Ingredients:
large egg 1
unsweetened applesauce 1 ½ cups
oat flour ⅓ cup
baking powder 2 tsp.
cinnamon ¾ tsp.

vegetable oil 2 Tbs.
whole wheat pastry flour 1 ⅔ cups
baking soda ¾ tsp.
nutmeg ½ tsp.

Preparation:
Beat together in medium bowl:
   1 large egg
   2 Tbs. vegetable oil
   1 ½ cups unsweetened applesauce

Combine in small bowl:
   1 ⅔ cups whole wheat pastry flour
   ⅓ cup oat flour
   ¾ tsp baking soda
   2 tsp. baking powder
   ½ tsp. nutmeg
   ¾ tsp. cinnamon
Add to applesauce mixture
Beat well

Spoon batter into greased muffin tins
Bake at 375° for 20 to 25 minutes

BLUEBERRY MUFFINS
12 muffins

Ingredients:
baking powder 2 ½ tsp.
salt ½ tsp.
egg 1
milk ⅓ cup

whole wheat pastry flour 1 ¾ cups
blueberries ¾ cup
orange juice ⅓ cup
vegetable oil ¼ cup

Preparation:
Combine in medium bowl:
1 ¾ cups whole wheat pastry flour
2 ½ tsp. baking powder
½ tsp. salt
¾ cup blueberries

Combine in small bowl:
1 egg, beaten
⅓ cup orange juice
⅓ cup milk
¼ cup vegetable oil

Add liquids to:
flour mixture
Stir until dry ingredients are moistened

Drop batter from tablespoon into greased muffin pans
Bake at 400° for about 25 minutes

LIGHT MUFFINS
6 muffins

Ingredients:

oat flour 1 cup	salt ⅛ tsp.
baking powder 2 ½ tsp.	eggs 2
unsweetened orange juice ¼ cup	butter 2 Tbs.

Preparation:
Combine in medium bowl:
1 cup oat flour
⅛ tsp. salt
2 ½ tsp baking powder
Combine in small bowl:
2 eggs, well beaten
¼ cup orange juice
2 Tbs. melted butter
Add to flour mixture and stir till smooth
Pour batter into oiled muffin tin
Bake at 425° for 25 minutes
Delicious with butter and fresh unsweetened applesauce

BRAN MUFFINS
12 muffins

Ingredients:

vegetable oil ¼ cup
unsweetened orange juice ⅓ cup
eggs 2
oats ¼ cup
baking powder 1 Tbs
Apples 1 cup (optional)
*frozen

*concentrated apple juice 2 Tbs
milk ⅓ cup
whole wheat pastry flour ¾ cup
unprocessed Bran 1 cup
salt ¼ tsp

Preparation:

Beat together until light and fluffy:
   ¼ cup vegetable oil
   2 Tbs. unsweetened concentrated apple juice

Blend in:
   ⅓ cup milk
   ⅓ cup unsweetened orange juice
   2 eggs

Combine and add to above mixture:
   ¾ cup whole wheat pastry flour
   ¼ cup oat flour
   1 cup unprocessed Bran
   1 Tbs. baking powder
   ¼ tsp. salt
Mix until just moistened

Optional:
Fold in:
   1 cup finely chopped apples
Pour batter into greased muffin tin
Bake at 400° for 15 - 20 minutes

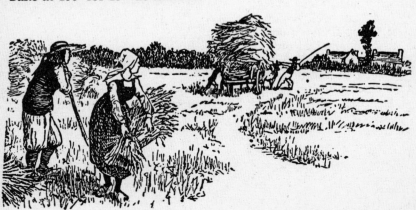

CRANBERRY MUFFINS
12 muffins

Ingredients:
raw cranberries 1 cup
oat flour ⅓ cup
salt ¼ tsp.
egg 1
sour milk or buttermilk ¾ cup
*frozen

*concentrated orange juice ⅓ cup
whole wheat pastry flour 1 ¾ cups
baking soda ¾ tsp.
*concentrated apple juice 2 Tbs.
vegetable oil 2 Tbs.

Preparation:
Combine in small bowl:
    1 cup raw, chopped cranberries
    ⅓ cup unsweetened concentrated orange juice

Combine in medium bowl:
    1 ¾ cups whole wheat pastry flour
    ⅓ cup oat flour
    ¼ tsp salt
    ¾ tsp. baking soda

Combine in small bowl:
    2 Tbs. unsweetened concentrated apple juice
    1 egg, beaten
    ¾ cup sour milk or buttermilk
    2 Tbs. vegetable oil

Add:
    liquids to flour mixture
Stir till mixed

Add:
    cranberries and juice
Mix gently

Spoon batter into greased muffins tin
Bake at 400° for 20 minutes

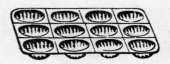

OAT MUFFINS

12 muffins or 1 8x8 in. square baking dish

Ingredients:

oat flour 2 ¼ cups
baking soda ¼ tsp.
egg 1
sour or buttermilk ¾ cup
apricots ⅓ cup (optional)

baking powder 2 tsp.
salt ½ tsp.
*concentrated orange juice 2 Tbs.
vegetable oil ¼ cup

*frozen

Preparation:

Combine:
2 ¼ cups oat flour
2 tsp. baking powder
¼ tsp. baking soda
½ tsp. salt

Combine and add to above:
1 well beaten egg
2 Tbs. unsweetened concentrated orange juice
¾ cup sour or buttermilk
¼ cup vegetable oil
⅓ cup chopped apricots (optional)
Stir quickly till dry ingredients are moistened

Pour batter into greased muffin tin or 8 in. square baking dish
Bake at 400° for 25 minutes, a little longer if using baking dish

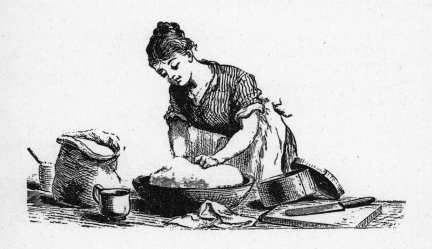

OATMEAL MUFFINS
12 Muffins

Ingredients:
rolled oats 1 cup
egg 1
vegetable oil ½ cup minus 1 Tbs.
baking powder 1 tsp
baking soda ½ tsp.

*frozen

sour milk 1 cup
*concentrated apple juice 2 Tbs.
soy flour 2 Tbs.
whole. wheat pastry flour ⅞ cup
salt ¼ tsp.

Preparation:
Soak for 1 hour in medium bowl:
    1 cup oats
In:
    1 cup sour milk **

Add and beat well:
    1 egg

Add and mix well:
    2 Tbs. concentrated apple juice
Add:
    ½ cup minus 1 Tbs. vegetable oil

Place in cup:
    2 Tbs. soy flour
    enough whole wheat pastry flour to make 1 cup

Combine in small bowl:
    flour mixture
    1 tsp. baking powder
    ½ tsp. baking soda
    ¼ tsp. salt
Add flour mixture to:
    liquids
Mix well

Pour batter into muffin pan, fill ⅔ full
Bake 15 to 20 minutes at 400°

**To make sour milk:
    put 1 Tbs. + 1 tsp. vinegar in cup, add enough milk to fill cup.

If you don't enjoy washing muffin pans, bake in a 10 x 6 x 2 in. baking
    dish for about 30 mins.

NICE THREE GRAIN MUFFINS
10-12 muffins

Ingredients:
soy flour ¼ cup
oat flour ⅓ cup
baking powder 3 tsp.
eggs 2
dried apricots ¼ cup (optional)

whole wheat pastry flour 1 ½ cups
salt ¼ tsp.
vegetable oil 5 tsp.
apple juice 1 cup

Preparation:
Combine in medium bowl:
    ¼ cup soy flour
    ⅓ cup oat flour
    1 ½ cups whole wheat pastry flour
    ¼ tsp. salt
    3 tsp. baking powder

Beat together in small bowl:
    5 tsp. vegetable oil
    2 eggs
    1 cup apple juice
Add to dry ingredients
Stir enough to moisten

Fold in:
    ¼ cup chopped, dried apricots (optional)
Spoon batter into oiled muffin tin
Bake at 400° for 15-20 minutes

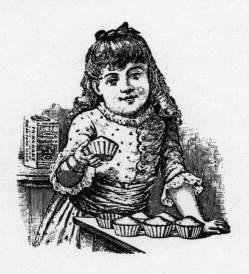

CRANBERRY NUT LOAF
1 loaf

Ingredients:

whole wheat pastry flour 1 cup
soy flour 1 Tbs.
baking soda ½ tsp.
vegetable oil 3 Tbs.
orange rind 1 Tbs.
*concentrated apple juice ¼ cup
walnuts ¾ cup

*frozen

oat flour 1 ¼ cups
baking powder 1 ¾ tsp.
salt ½ tsp.
orange juice ½ cup
egg 1
*concentrated pineapple juice ¼ cup
fresh cranberries 1 cup

Preparation:

Sift together in large bowl:
  1 cup whole wheat flour
  1 ¼ cups oat flour
  1 Tbs. soy flour
  1 ¾ tsp. baking powder
  ½ tsp. baking soda
  ½ tsp salt

Combine in small bowl:
  3 Tbs. vegetable oil
  ½ cup orange juice
  1 Tbs. orange rind
  1 egg, beaten
  ¼ cup frozen concentrated apple juice
  ¼ cup frozen concentrated pineapple juice
Pour into dry ingredients

Mix just enough to dampen

Fold in:
  ¾ cup chopped walnuts
  1 cup chopped fresh cranberries

Spoon into 9" x 5" x 3" pan, spread corners & sides slightly higher than center
Bake at 350° about 1 hour till crust golden brown and toothpick comes out clean.

BANANA NUT LOAF
1 loaf

Ingredients:

vegetable oil ½ cup
*concentrated apple juice ¼ cup
ripe bananas 3 medium size
whole wheat pastry flour 1 cup
Ezekiel flour ¼ cup
wheat germ ½ cup
baking powder 2 tsp.
walnuts ¾ cup

*concentrated pineapple juice ¼ cup
vanilla 1 ¼ tsp.
eggs 2
oat flour ¼ cup
soy flour 1 Tbs
salt ¼ tsp.
cinnamon ¾ tsp.

*frozen

Prepartion:

Combine in large bowl:
  ½ cup vegetable oil
  ¼ cup concentrated pineapple juice
  ¼ cup concentrated apple juice

Add:
  1 ¼ tsp. vanilla
  3 smashed medium size ripe bananas
  2 eggs, beaten
Mix well

Combine and add to above:
  1 cup whole wheat pastry flour
  ¼ cup oat flour, sifted
  ¼ cup Ezekiel flour
  1 Tbs. soy flour
  ½ cup wheat germ
  ¼ tsp. salt
  2 tsp. baking powder
  ¾ tsp. cinnamon
  ¾ cup chopped walnuts
Stir only until well mixed

Place in well greased 9" x 5" x 3" pan
Bake at 325° for 1 hr. & 15 mins. or until well browned and crusty

BEVERAGES

Fruit juices are very good if you drink them in small portions and slowly. You can find many unsweetened fruit juices in your health food store and a few in your local grocery store.

Depending on how well you can tolerate fruit juices, you may want to dilute the juices with water or carbonated water to decrease their concentration of natural sugar. These juices alone or in combination with each other afford you a variety of beverages to enjoy. But please remember, you should drink only a small amount (3-5 oz.) of juice at any one time and be sure to keep water as your main beverage (6-8 glasses a day).

A few brand names of unsweetened fruit juices are, After The Fall, Apple & Eve, Dole, Nice & Natural, R. W. Knudsen, and Red cheek. But you must always read labels for changes.

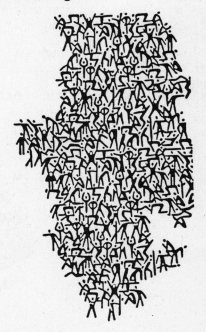

LIMEADE
serves 2

Ingredients, chilled:
fresh lime juice ½ cup   *concentrated orange juice 1 Tbs.
carbonated water 1 ½ cups

*frozen

Preparation:
Mix together:
½ cup fresh lime juice
1 Tbs. concentrated orange juice
1 ½ cups carbonated water
Serve over crushed ice with slice of lime on glass edge

May use lemon juice in place of lime

HOT SPICED CIDER
serves 2

Ingredients:
cider 2 cups   cinnamon-spice herb tea 3 bags

Preparation:
Heat in small saucepan over moderate heat:
2 cups cider
Add:
3 bags cinnamon-spice herb tea
Turn off heat
Steep 5-10 minutes
Serve sprinkled with cinnamon or nutmeg

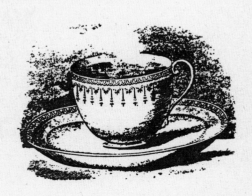

FRUIT JUICE DELIGHT
serves 8-10

Ingredients, chilled:
Fresh orange juice 1 cup
lemon juice ⅓ cup
apple cranberry juice ice cubes

unsweetened apple-cranberry juice 4 cups
carbonated water 28 oz.

Preparation:
Combine:
  1 cup fresh orange juice
  4 cups unsweetened apple-cranberry juice
  ⅓ cup lemon juice

Gently add:
  28 oz. carbonated water
Stir gently
Serve over ice cubes made with apple cranberry juice

FRUIT PUNCH
serves 6-8

Ingredients, chilled:
unsweetened orange juice 3 cups
carbonated water 1 quart
fresh whole strawberries

unsweetened pineapple juice 3 cups
frozen unsweetened strawberries 10 oz.
orange slices

Preparation:
Blend in blender:
  3 cups unsweetened orange juice
  3 cups unsweetened pineapple juice
  10 oz. thawed, unsweetened strawberries
Add to:
  1 quart carbonated water

Place in ring mold:
  whole strawberries
  orange slices

Add:
  4 cups punch
Freeze
Chill remaining punch
Serve from bowl with ice ring floating in punch

Listed below are vegetables and fruits with their percentage of carbohydrate content. Do not eat two items from the 15% list in one meal. Remember, carbohydrates convert to sugar (glucose).

The following list of foods is but a small example of how specific you must be when dealing with which foods to eat. This concept is explained in much greater detail in The Low Blood Sugar Handbook. (See order form in back of book.)

Vegetables

3% to 5% Carbohydrates—no limit on amount or frequency.

bamboo shoots	endive	parsley
beet greens	escarole	peppers, sweet
celery	fennel	pickles, dill & sour
chicory	kale	poke
Chinese cabbage	lettuce	radishes
chives	mushrooms	spinach
collard greens	mustard greens	turnip greens
cucumbers	olives	watercress

6% to 9% Carbohydrates—no limit on amount or frequency.

asparagus	chard	peppers, hot
bamboo shoots	dandelion greens	pimentos
bean sprouts	eggplant	sauerkraut
beans—green & wax	kohlrabi	summer squash
broccoli	okra	tomato
cabbage	onions	turnips
cauliflower	peas, edible pods	zucchini

10% to 14% Carbohydrates—have vegetables from this list only once per day, be watchful of quantity.

artichoke—globe	celeriac	soybeans
beets	chervil	soybean sprouts
Brussels sprouts	leeks	squash, winter
carrots	rutabaga	tomato puree
		water chestnuts

15% + Carbohydrates—Have only a small serving. Do not eat two of these vegetables in the same day or with bread, gravy, or 10% or 15% fruit.

artichoke, Jerusalem	parsnips	split peas
kidney beans	peas	

Vegetables to eat seldom and in very small portion

black eyed peas	lentils	potatoes
corn & corn products	lima beans	sweet potatoes
dried beans & peas	navy beans	yams

Vegetables to avoid

blackbeans	hominy	sweet relish
garbanzos (ckickpeas)	sweet pickles	pinto beans

Fruits

It is well recognized that fruit is an important part of your nutritional and aesthetic desires. However, since fruit is very high in natural sugar (simple carbohydrate), some LBS sufferers cannot tolerate any fruit, others can handle a small amount infrequently, while some can tolerate a small amount daily.

Guess who is the only person in the world who can tell how much fruit you are able to eat? You guessed it, only you can determine the frequency and amount of fruit you are able to eat. It will depend on how you feel and function on the day of and/or a day or two after eating fruit. If symptoms return, fruit should be one of the first items consdered to be the cause; therefore eat fruit of lower carbohydrate concentration or eat less fruit or stop eating fruit completely.

No matter what position you take, every once in a while you should consider not eating fruit and drinking juices for a two or three week period and see if your brain clears up (the clouds go away) in how it and you are functioning (less anxiety and/or mood swings). During this period you may also want to cut back or stop eating all starchy foods (breads, pasta, rice, potatoes, corn and other grains).

5% to 9% Carbohydrates—1 cup serving

avocado	guava	strawberries
cantaloupe	loquat	watermelon
grapefruit		

10% to 14% Carbohydrates—½ cup serving

applesauce, unsweetened	gooseberries	orange
apricots, fresh	honeydew melon	papaya
blackberries	kiwi	peach
blueberries	lemon	pineapple
boysenberries	lime	pomegranate
casaba melon	lychee	quince
cranberries, unsweetened	mulberries	raspberries
	muskmelon	tangerines
	nectarines	

15% + Carbohydrates—do not eat daily and eat only a very small portion with caution in mind; do not eat with other fruits or with 15% vegetables or bread.

apples	elderberries	pears
cherries	kumquat	persimmons
coconut, fresh	loganberries	plums
currants, black	mango	youngberries
dewberries	passion fruit	

Fruits to eat seldom and in very small portion

banana	grapes

Fruits to avoid

dates	figs	plantain
dried fruit	fruits canned in syrup	prunes

Beverages:

Healthwise it is recommended that you drink 6 to 8 eight ounce glasses of water a day. The cells in your body need moisture to be healthy. This water is not the water that is in any other beverage, it is plain water.

Even though herb teas have no caffeine, you should be wary of them because they may have a natural substance which is detrimental and also they may put you back in the habit of desiring or even drinking regular tea and coffee.

0% to 4% Carbohydrates

clear broth	seltzer water	water
herb tea		

5% to 9% Carbohydrates—½ cup per day

milk	tomato juice	vegetable juice
sauerkraut juice		

10% to 14% Carbohydrates—½ cup per day

apple juice	grapefruit juice	pomegranate juice
blackberry juice	orange juice	tangerine juice
carrot juice		

15% + Carbohydrates—½ cup per day

apricot nectar	pear nectar	raspberry juice
loganberry juice	pineapple juice	

Beverages to avoid

alcohol	grape juice	soft drinks
cocoa	ovaltine	strong tea
coffee	papaya juice	excessive amounts of any
colas	postum	fruit or vegetable juice.
chocolate	prune juice	

Other Foods To Avoid—items that have any type of sugar and/or artificial sweetener, cornstarch or MSG added.

Breads, bread products, crackers and pasta—made with white flour and/or sugar

Meats—all lunch meats and cold cuts; usually have some form of sugar and fillers, read labels carefully.

Snack food

corn chips	popcorn	potato chips

Desserts—anything made with white flour and/or sugar

Sweets

candy	jam	molasses
caramel	jelly	sugar
chewing gum	malt	syrup
honey	marmalade	

INDEX

The authors encourage you to share with them any questions or insights you may have. A great amount of work still needs to be done in the study of low blood sugar and its effects. If an answer is desired, include a stamped, self addressed envelope. Please write to us c/o:

Franklin Publishers
P.O. Box 1338
Bryn Mawr, Pa. 19010

ORDER YOUR COPY(S) TODAY!

___copy(s)___ THE LOW BLOOD SUGAR HANDBOOK (Revised edition) $12.95

___copy(s)___ THE LOW BLOOD SUGAR COOKBOOK $12.95

___copy(s)___ THE LOW BLOOD SUGAR CASSETTE (1 hour) .... $ 9.95

___copy(s)___ COMPOSITION OF FOODS BOOKLET .... $ 4.50

___copy(s)___ CHOLESTEROL LOWERING AND CONTROLLING
3 WEEK PLAN: HANDBOOK & COOKBOOK $12.95

Send check or money order to: **Franklin Publishers, Box 1338, Bryn Mawr, PA 19010.**
For total order, include $2.00 for postage and handling or $3.00 for 1st class postage
and handling.   PA residents, include state sales tax.

Orders outside of U.S. must be paid in U.S. dollars with a Postal Money Order.

Send to:

Mr./Ms. _____
(Print or type)

Address_____

City_____ State_____ Zip_____

Phone number _____

Price subject to change without notice.

ORDER YOUR COPY(S) TODAY!

___copy(s)___ THE LOW BLOOD SUGAR HANDBOOK (Revised edition) $12.95

___copy(s)___ THE LOW BLOOD SUGAR COOKBOOK $12.95

___copy(s)___ THE LOW BLOOD SUGAR CASSETTE (1 hour) .... $ 9.95

___copy(s)___ COMPOSITION OF FOODS BOOKLET .... $ 4.50

___copy(s)___ CHOLESTEROL LOWERING AND CONTROLLING
3 WEEK PLAN: HANDBOOK & COOKBOOK $12.95

Send check or money order to: **Franklin Publishers, Box 1338, Bryn Mawr, PA 19010.**
For total order, include $2.00 for postage and handling or $3.00 for 1st class postage
and handling.   PA residents, include state sales tax.

Orders outside of U.S. must be paid in U.S. dollars with a Postal Money Order.

Send to:

Mr./Ms. _____
(Print or type)

Address_____

City_____ State_____ Zip_____

Phone number _____

Price subject to change without notice.

ORDER YOUR COPY(S) TODAY!

___ THE LOW BLOOD SUGAR HANDBOOK (Revised edition) $12.95
copy(s)

___ THE LOW BLOOD SUGAR COOKBOOK $12.95
copy(s)

___ THE LOW BLOOD SUGAR CASSETTE (1 hour) . . . . $ 9.95
copy(s)

___ COMPOSITION OF FOODS BOOKLET . . . . $ 4.50
copy(s)

___ CHOLESTEROL LOWERING AND CONTROLLING
copy(s) 3 WEEK PLAN: HANDBOOK & COOKBOOK $12.95

Send check or money order to: **Franklin Publishers, Box 1338, Bryn Mawr, PA 19010.**
For total order, include $2.00 for postage and handling or $3.00 for 1st class postage
and handling.   PA residents, include state sales tax.

Orders outside of U.S. must be paid in U.S. dollars with a Postal Money Order.

Send to:

Mr./Ms. _____
          (Print or type)

Address_____

City_____ State_____ Zip_____

Phone number _____
                    Price subject to change without notice.

ORDER YOUR COPY(S) TODAY!

___ THE LOW BLOOD SUGAR HANDBOOK (Revised edition) $12.95
copy(s)

___ THE LOW BLOOD SUGAR COOKBOOK $12.95
copy(s)

___ THE LOW BLOOD SUGAR CASSETTE (1 hour) . . . . $ 9.95
copy(s)

___ COMPOSITION OF FOODS BOOKLET . . . . $ 4.50
copy(s)

___ CHOLESTEROL LOWERING AND CONTROLLING
copy(s) 3 WEEK PLAN: HANDBOOK & COOKBOOK $12.95

Send check or money order to: **Franklin Publishers, Box 1338, Bryn Mawr, PA 19010.**
For total order, include $2.00 for postage and handling or $3.00 for 1st class postage
and handling.   PA residents, include state sales tax.

Orders outside of U.S. must be paid in U.S. dollars with a Postal Money Order.

Send to:

Mr./Ms. _____
          (Print or type)

Address_____

City_____ State_____ Zip_____

Phone number _____
                    Price subject to change without notice.

To order, send note or copy of order form with payment

ABOUT THE AUTHORS

Edward and Patricia Krimmel and their son, Charles, live in the western suburbs of Philadelphia, Pa.

Patricia and Edward Krimmel are medical researchers and writers who have a special aptitude and spirit for relating very well to those trying to solve health problems. Because of their backgrounds, they are especially well equipped to write and design books dealing with solutions rather than simply talking about the problem. They are the authors of two other books; *The Low Blood Sugar Handbook* and *The Cholesterol Lowering and Controlling Handbook and Cookbook.*

Pat has her BSN from the University of Pennsylvania, has worked in childbirth education, public health and has been Maternal and Infant Care Coordinator at the Medical College of Pennsylvania.

Ed has his degree in Social Science from Saint Joseph's University, is Director of Help, The Institute For Body Chemistry, and does nutritional counseling.

Ed and Pat coordinate self help meetings for those interested in body chemistry. They lecture extensively at colleges, health fairs and are guests on talk shows.

For over 15 years they have been helping others learn about low blood sugar. Their book, The Low Blood Sugar Handbook, is heralded as the most complete and comprehensive book on the subject, truly the book of solutions!

NEWSLETTER! NEWSLETTER! NEWSLETTER!

How would you like to receive current information in the world of body chemistry, nutrition, biochemistry, LBS, PMS, well-being, and so on? Send a self addressed, stamped envelope to: Franklin Publishers, Box 1338, Bryn Mawr, PA 19010.

COMMUNITY SUPPORT GROUP

If you are interested in having a self help support group started in your community or locating one already established, mail us your name, address and phone number. Explain your need and desire. Mail to: Franklin Publishers, Box 1338, Bryn Mawr, PA 19010. Include self address, stamped envelope.